# World Clinics

Pulmonary & Critical Care Medicine

## Respiratory Critical Care

# World Clinics

Pulmonary & Critical Care Medicine

## Respiratory Critical Care

*Editor-in-Chief*
**Surinder K Jindal** MD FAMS FNCCP FCCP

*Guest Editor*
**Randeep Guleria** MD DM

January 2016  Volume 4  Number 1

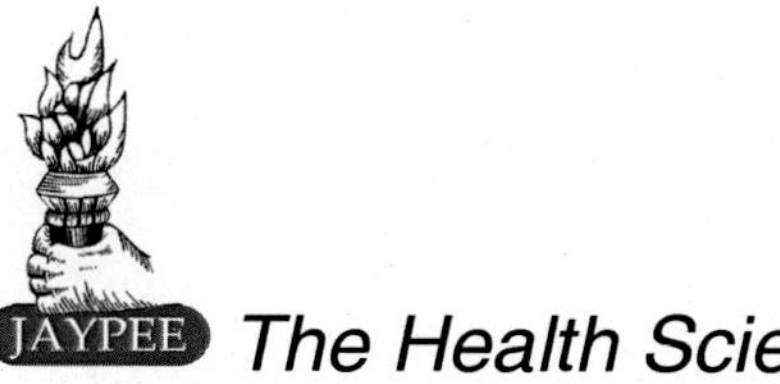

**JAYPEE** *The Health Sciences Publisher*

New Delhi | London | Philadelphia | Panama

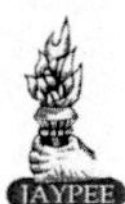

**Jaypee Brothers Medical Publishers (P) Ltd**

**Headquarters**

Jaypee Brothers Medical Publishers (P) Ltd
4838/24, Ansari Road, Daryaganj
New Delhi 110 002, India
Phone: +91-11-43574357
Fax: +91-11-43574314
Email: jaypee@jaypeebrothers.com

**Overseas Offices**

J.P. Medical Ltd
83 Victoria Street, London
SW1H 0HW (UK)
Phone: +44-2031708910
Fax: +02-03-0086180
Email: info@jpmedpub.com

Jaypee Medical Inc
325 Chestnul Street
Suite 412, Philadelphia, PA 19106, USA
Phone: +1 267-519-9789
Email: support@jpmedus.com

Jaypee Brothers Medical Publishers (P) Ltd
Bhotahity, Kathmandu, Nepal
Phone: +977-9741283608
Email: Kathmandu@jaypeebrothers.com

Jaypee-Highlights Medical Publishers Inc
City of Knowledge, Bld. 237, Clayton
Panama City, Panama
Phone: +1 507-301-0496
Fax: +1 507-301-0499
Email: cservice@jphmedical.com

Jaypee Brothers Medical Publishers (P) Ltd
17/1-B Babar Road, Block-B, Shaymali
Mohammadpur, Dhaka-1207
Bangladesh
Mobile: +08801912003485
Email: jaypeedhaka@gmail.com

Website: www.jaypeebrothers.com
Website: www.jaypeedigital.com



Cover images: (*Left*) Window of opportunity to intervene with targeting edema in first phase, anti-inflammatory therapies in second phase and antifibrotic strategies in third phase. *Courtesy:* Deepak Talwar, Arjun Khanna. (*Right*) Computed tomography angiography showing a massive pulmonary embolism. *Courtesy:* Devasahayam J Christopher, Richa Gupta.

WORLD CLINICS Pulmonary and Critical Care Medicine: Respiratory Critical Care
January 2016, Volume 4, Number 1
ISSN: 2319-1260
ISBN: 978-93-85999-61-1

Printed at Replika Press Pvt. Ltd.

Printed in India

# Contributors

## Editor-in-Chief

Surinder K Jindal MD FAMS FNCCP FCCP
Medical Director
Jindal Clinics
Chandigarh, India

## Guest Editor

Randeep Guleria MD DM
Professor and Head
Department of Pulmonary Medicine and Sleep Disorders
All India Institute of Medical Sciences
New Delhi, India

## Contributing Authors

Ashutosh N Aggarwal MD DM
Professor
Department of Pulmonary Medicine
Postgraduate Institute of Medical Education and Research
Chandigarh, India

Ritesh Agarwal MD DM
Additional Professor
Department of Pulmonary Medicine
Postgraduate Institute of Medical Education and Research
Chandigarh, India

Dhruva Chaudhry MD DNB DM FICP FICCM
Senior Professor and Head
Department of Pulmonary and Critical Care Medicine
Pt BD Sharma Post Graduate Institute of Medical Sciences
Rohtak, Haryana, India

Rajesh Chawla MD FCCP FCCM
Senior Consultant
Department of Respiratory Medicine, Critical Care, and Sleep Medicine
Indraprastha Apollo Hospitals
New Delhi, India

Devasahayam J Christopher BSc DTCD DNB FICS FRCP FCCP
Professor and Head
Department of Pulmonary Medicine
Christian Medical College
Vellore, Tamil Nadu, India

Raja Dhar MD MRCP MSc CCT FCCP
Consultant Pulmonologist and Intensivist
Head, Department of Respiratory Medicine
Fortis Hospital
Kolkata, West Bengal, India

Sahajal Dhooria MD DM
Assistant Professor
Department of Pulmonary Medicine
Postgraduate Institute of Medical Education and Research
Chandigarh, India

Richa Gupta MD FCCP
Professor
Department of Pulmonary Medicine
Christian Medical College and Hospital
Vellore, Tamil Nadu, India

Vijay Hadda MD
Assistant Professor
Department of Pulmonary Medicine and Sleep Disorders
All India Institute of Medical Sciences
New Delhi, India

Aditya Jindal MBBS DNB DM FCCP
Consultant Pulmonologist, Jindal Clinics
Centre for Interventional Pulmonology and Sleep Medicine
Chandigarh, India

Deven Juneja DNB FNB EDIC FCCP IFCCM FCCM
Senior Consultant and Incharge
Department of Critical Care and Emergency Medicine
Shri Balaji Action Medical Institute
New Delhi, India

Arjun Khanna MD DM
Consultant
Department of Pulmonary and Critical Care Medicine
Metro Center for Respiratory Diseases, Metro Hospital and Heart Institute
Noida, Uttar Pradesh, India

Karan Madan MD DM
Assistant Professor
Department of Pulmonary Medicine and Sleep Disorders
All India Institute of Medical Sciences
New Delhi, India

Saurabh Mittal MD
Senior Resident
Department of Pulmonary Medicine and Sleep Disorders
All India Institute of Medical Sciences
New Delhi, India

Nicholas Raush MD
Housestaff Physician
Department of Internal Medicine
University of Alabama at Birmingham
Birmingham, Alabama, United States

Inderpaul S Sehgal MD DNB DM
Assistant Professor
Department of Pulmonary Medicine
Postgraduate Institute of Medical Education and Research
Chandigarh, India

Navneet Singh MD DM FACP FCCP FICS
Associate Professor
Department of Pulmonary Medicine
Postgraduate Institute of Medical Education and Research
Chandigarh, India

Deepak Talwar MD DM
Director and Chair
Metro Center for Respiratory Diseases, Metro Hospital and Heart Institute
Noida, Uttar Pradesh, India

Jennifer Trevor MD
Assistant Professor
Department of Pulmonary, Allergy, and Critical Care Medicine
University of Alabama at Birmingham
Birmingham, Alabama, United States

John P Willoughby MD BS
Housestaff Physician
Department of Internal Medicine
University of Alabama at Birmingham
Birmingham, Alabama, United States

# Contents

# Editorial

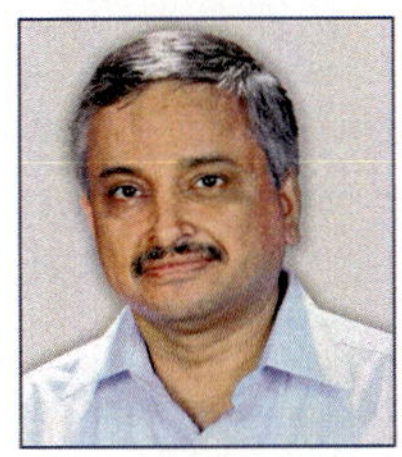

**Randeep Guleria** MD DM
*Guest Editor*

Intensive care is a relatively new super specialty that has shown major advances in the last two decades. From initially being an area where better monitoring was done for very sick patients, it has now become an aggressive field with interventions, defined treatment strategies, and better multispecialty care. Research in this area over the last few years has changed the way we are practicing critical care today. Respiratory care in many ways forms the core of critical care medicine. It is for this reason that many pulmonologists all over the world are also critical care specialist. It is becoming increasingly important for pulmonologists, intensivists, and internists to keep abreast with newer developments in the area of critical care medicine. This issue is aimed at trying to provide some basic and advanced knowledge in key areas of critical care medicine.

Respiratory support mainly with invasive ventilation is usually the area around which most patients' management revolves. We have now a better understanding of the "good and bad" of mechanical ventilation and this has guided ventilatory management over the last few years. From a high tidal volume strategy, we have now routinely come to accept a strategy of low tidal volume in most of our ventilated patients with an underlying lung disease.

One area where mortality continues to be high is acute respiratory distress syndrome (ARDS). The last decade has seen a number of positive and negative studies in this area. Well-conducted study by the Acute Respiratory Distress Syndrome Network group has provided evidence based ventilator and critical care management strategies for patients with ARDS. Well-defined protocols for the management of ARDS have been developed and are used in most intensive care units (ICUs). Low tidal volume strategy is now a well-established method for ventilation in these patients. Similarly, data on a conservative fluid strategy for ARDS and thereby keeping the lungs relatively dry is also emerging. High frequency ventilation which was initially thought to be useful has been shown to be of no use and is currently not recommended. Prone position ventilation may be helpful in patients with refractory hypoxemia although it is difficult to perform in many ICUs. Similarly, more recent data, especially after the H1N1 pandemic, suggest that extracorporeal membrane oxygenation may also be a useful modality if available in patients with ARDS and refractory hypoxemia. Noninvasive ventilation has also emerged as a very effective modality especially in chronic obstructive pulmonary disease patients. Recent studies on noninvasive ventilation have helped to set established guidelines as to where this mode of ventilation will be helpful and where it is contraindicated. As technology has advanced, newer ventilators with microchips have been developed providing additional modes of ventilation. How effective these are in providing better ventilation and help in weaning still needs to be established and more research is needed in this area.

Sepsis is another area where there have been a lot of recent articles which have looked at treatment strategies. Early goal directed therapy (EGDT) has become almost standard of care for the management of septic shock. More recent studies have challenged many aspects of EGDT showing that although we need to follow these principles a strict protocol-based regimen may not be that important in decreasing mortality. Similarly, tight glycemic control is no longer important in critical care and so is the case with blood transfusion unless the hemoglobin is less than 7 g/dL.

Many patients admitted in the ICU have exacerbation of their chronic obstructive lung disease. Managing these patients who have type 2 respiratory failure is another challenge. It is important to understand the basic pathophysiology behind this disease and thereby be clear on the utility of both invasive and noninvasive ventilation in these patients. Similarly, deep vein thrombosis and pulmonary embolism remains underdiagnosed in most ICUs. The routine use of ultrasound in the ICUs is changing all this. With regular screening of the leg veins at the bedside and basic bedside echocardiography in the intensive care the early diagnosis of deep vein thrombosis and pulmonary embolism has become possible. It is therefore imperative that all physicians working in the intensive care area become well versed in the use of ultrasound in pulmonary and critical care. Ultrasound in critical care is useful not only in helping in various interventions but is also a valuable beside tool for the diagnosis of various medical emergencies like pneumothorax, pneumonia, effusions, fluid overload, and, as already mentioned, pulmonary embolism.

Also prevention and management of infection that occur in the intensive care is of paramount importance. Infection itself can be the reason for ICU care due to shock and multiorgan failure. Hospital-acquired infection occurs is common in most ICUs and is a major cause of morbidity and mortality. Taking adequate steps to prevent infection in the ICU is therefore an important area which gets neglected in most ICUs. Similarly, the basic principle of medicine "first do no harm" is all the more important in an ICU setting. Many ICU-related complications kill the patients rather than the disease itself. It is, therefore, essential to weigh the risk versus benefit of many interventions we do in the ICU.

Finally, critical care also needs a more humane and compassionate face. In an ICU setting, where the patient is isolated from his relatives and doctors attending to him are all wearing masks and gown, there is a need for intensivists to understand the patient's fears and anxieties. Also, there is a need to critically look at the current cost of treatment in the ICU and work on strategies to decrease this cost of treatment in the ICU. In India, the cost of treatment in the ICU is currently very high and we need to develop innovative and effective means to manage our patients in the critical care setting in a cost effective manner.

**Randeep Guleria** MD DM
Professor and Head
Department of Pulmonary Medicine and Sleep Disorders
All India Institute of Medical Sciences
New Delhi, India

# Abbreviations

| | |
|---|---|
| 2D | Two-dimensional |
| ABCD | Airway, Breathing, Circulation, Drugs and Decontamination |
| ABG | Arterial blood gas |
| ACI | Acute critical illness |
| ACMV | Assist/control mode ventilation |
| ACOS | Asthma-COPD overlap syndrome |
| AECC | American-European Consensus Conference |
| AF | Atrial fibrillation |
| AIDS | Acquired immunodeficiency syndrome |
| ALI | Acute lung injury |
| APACHE II | Acute Physiology and Chronic Health Evaluation II |
| APTT | Activated partial thromboplastin time |
| ARDS | Adult respiratory distress syndrome |
| ARDSNet | Acute Respiratory Distress Syndrome Network |
| ARF | Acute respiratory failure |
| ASV | Adaptive servo-ventilation |
| ATC | Automatic tube compensation |
| AVP | Arginine vasopressin |
| BD | Twice a day |
| BMI | Body mass index |
| BMR | Basal metabolic rate |
| BNP | Brain natriuretic peptide |
| BP | Blood pressure |
| BPPV | Bilevel positive pressure ventilation |
| cAG | Corrected anion gap |
| $CaO_2$ | Arterial oxygen content |
| CAP | Community-acquired pneumonia |
| CCI | Chronic critical illness |
| Ccw | Chest wall compliance |
| CDC | Centers for Disease Control and Prevention |
| Cdyn | Dynamic compliance |
| CESAR | Conventional Care versus Extracorporeal Support in Adult Respiratory Failure |
| CI | Confidence interval |
| CL | Lung compliance |
| CLT | Cuff leak test |
| CMV | Control mode ventilation |
| CNS | Central nervous system |
| CO | Carbon monoxide |
| $CO_2$ | Carbon dioxide |
| COPD | Chronic obstructive pulmonary disease |
| CPAP | Continuous positive airway pressure |
| CROP | Compliance, rate, oxygenation, pressure |
| CRP | C-reactive protein |
| Cstat | Static compliance |
| CT | Computed tomography |
| CTPA | Computed tomography pulmonary arteriography |
| CUS | Compression ultrasonography |
| DVT | Deep vein thrombosis |
| EAdi | Electrical activity of the diaphragm |
| ECG | Electrocardiogram |
| Echo | Echocardiography |
| ECMO | Extracorporeal membrane oxygenation |
| EMA | European Medicines Agency |
| EPAP | Expiratory positive airway pressure |
| ESBL | Extended-spectrum beta-lactamases |
| FDA | Food and Drug Administration |
| $FiO_2$ | Fraction of inspired oxygen |
| GABA | Gamma-aminobutyric acid |

| | |
|---|---|
| $H_2SO_4$ | Sulfuric acid |
| HAI | Hospital-acquired infection |
| Hb | Hemoglobin |
| HCl | Hydrochloric acid |
| $HCO_3^-$ | Bicarbonate |
| HFOV | High frequency oscillatory ventilation |
| HIT | Heparin-induced thrombocytopenia |
| HR | Heart rate |
| ICU | Intensive care unit |
| IgA | Immunoglobulin A |
| IgG | Immunoglobulin G |
| IL | Interleukin |
| IMV | Intermittent mandatory ventilation |
| INR | International normalized ratio |
| IPAP | Inspiratory positive airway pressure |
| IQR | Interquartile range |
| IV | Intravenous |
| IVC | Inferior vena caval |
| LMWH | Low molecular weight heparin; |
| LTOT | Long-term oxygen therapy |
| MAP | Mean airway pressure |
| MDCT | Multi-detector CT |
| MDI | Metered-dose inhaler |
| MDMA | 3,4-methylenedioxy-methamphetamine |
| MODS | Multiple organ dysfunction syndrome |
| MRSA | Methicillin-resistant *Staphylococcus aureus* |
| NAC | N-acetylcysteine |
| NAPQI | N-acetyl-p-benzoquinone imine |
| NAVA | Neurally adjusted ventilatory assist |
| NEAP | Net endogenous acid production |
| NIH | National Institutes of Health |
| NIPPV | Noninvasive positive pressure ventilation |
| NIV | Noninvasive ventilation |
| NMB | Neuromuscular blockade |
| NMBA | Nondepolarizing neuromuscular blocking agent |

| | |
|---|---|
| NOAC | Newer oral anticoagulant |
| NSAID | Nonsteroidal anti-inflammatory drug |
| OCL | Organochlorine |
| OCP | Oral contraceptive pill |
| OD | Once a day |
| OHS | Obesity hypoventilation syndrome |
| OP | Organophosphate |
| OR | Odds ratio |
| OSA | Obstructive sleep apnea |
| OSCILLATE | Oscillation for Acute Respiratory Distress Syndrome Treated Early |
| PACI | Prolonged acute critical illness |
| $PaCO_2$ | Arterial partial pressure of carbon dioxide |
| $PACO_2$ | Alveolar carbon dioxide content |
| $PAO_2$ | Alveolar oxygen content |
| $PaO_2$ | Partial pressure of arterial oxygen |
| PAV | Proportional assist ventilation |
| PBW | Predict body weight |
| PC-CMV | Pressure-controlled continuous mandatory ventilation |
| $PCO_2$ | Partial pressure of carbon dioxide |
| PC-SIMV | Pressure-controlled synchronized intermittent mandatory ventilation |
| PCV | Pressure control ventilation |
| PE | Pulmonary embolism |
| PEEP | Positive end-expiratory pressure |
| PEFR | Peak expiratory flow rate |
| Pes | Esophageal pressure |
| PImax | Maximum inspiratory pressure |
| $PiO_2$ | Total amount of inspired oxygen |
| PIOPED II | Prospective Investigation of Pulmonary Embolism Diagnosis II |
| Ppeak | Peak pressure |
| Ppl | Pleural pressure |
| Pplat | Plateau pressure |
| PS | Pressure support |

| | |
|---|---|
| PSV | Pressure support ventilation |
| QUIAC | Quality Use of Antimicrobials in Intensive Care |
| RBC | Red blood cell |
| RCI | Recovery from critical illness |
| RCT | Randomized controlled trial |
| REE | Resting energy expenditure |
| RNAE | Renal net acid excretion |
| RR | Respiratory rate |
| RSBI | Rapid shallow breathing index |
| SBP | Systolic blood pressure |
| SBT | Spontaneous breathing trial |
| SFT | Skinfold thickness |
| SIMV | Synchronized intermittent mandatory ventilation |
| SSC | Surviving Sepsis Campaign |
| TEE | Total energy expenditure |
| THA | Total hip arthroplasty |
| TKA | Total knee arthroplasty |
| UFH | Unfractionated heparin |
| UTI | Urinary tract infection |
| VALI | Ventilator-associated lung injury |
| VAP | Ventilator-associated pneumonia |
| VCV | Volume-controlled ventilation |
| VKA | Vitamin K antagonist |
| VRE | vancomycin-resistant enterococcus |
| VT | Tidal volume |
| VTe | Expired tidal volume |
| VTE | Venous thromboembolism |
| VTi | Inspired tidal volume |

World Clin Pulm Crit Care Med. 2016;4(1):1-9.

# Evolution and the Core of Critical Care

*Randeep Guleria MD DM, Vijay Hadda MD

Department of Pulmonary Medicine and Sleep Disorders, All India Institute of Medical Sciences
New Delhi, India

## ABSTRACT

Critical care which consists of care of a cohort of severely ill patients in closely monitored environment and providing support to failing organ/s to maintain physiological normalcy with the underlying disease being treated is relatively new specialty of medicine which has evolved, like other specialties, over last five decades or so. The evolution has occurred in term of setting of critical care, use of technology, understanding of pathophysiology of various diseases, utility of some of the old "standard of care" therapeutic interventions, and some newer therapeutic interventions. Many of these were possible due to collaboration of various international organizations working in the field of critical care. This article summarizes the journey of evolution and modernization of critical care along with few challenges in this field.

## INTRODUCTION

Critical care is relatively new specialty of medicine which has evolved, like other specialties, over the last 5 decades or so.[1] Defining or compartmentalizing critical care to a particular organ may be difficult. It consists of care of a cohort of severely ill patients in a closely monitored environment and providing support to failing organ(s) to maintain physiological normalcy with the underlying disease treated. Modern days critical care involve sophisticated equipments, such as advanced type of ventilators, infusion pumps, gadgets for noninvasive monitoring of multiple vital variables, bedside ultrasound machine providing instant imaging, facility to provide extracorporeal membrane oxygenation, etc.[2] When we consider all these

---

*Corresponding author
*Email:* randeepguleria2002@yahoo.com

and look back, one can clearly see the technological advances in this field. Along with technological advancement, there has been better understanding of the pathophysiology of the diseases and disease mechanisms.[2] With this improvement in both technology and understanding, the field of critical care has slowly but definitely evolved. Considering the fact that this evolution took decades to reach current modern day care, it is clear that it will keep on evolving.

This article will highlight some the important aspects of the critical care and their evolution to present status and future.

## EVOLUTION OF INTENSIVE CARE UNIT

Many of us think that critical care is a modern concept, however, organ supporting dates back to thousands of years. Some of the modern day practices like tracheostomy have been described by Egyptian as early as 1500 BC.[3] Approximately thousand years later, Hippocrates mentioned organ support in the form of cannulating the airway to allow the air to be drawn into the lungs. Florence Nightingale was the pioneer of highlighting the importance of geographical area for care of more seriously ill.[4] During Crimean war in the 1850s, she kept more serious patients near the nursing station so that they could be monitored more closely. Subsequently, in 1923, at Johns Hopkins Hospital, Baltimore, USA, a specialized three bed unit was established for care of more seriously postoperative neurosurgical patients.[5,6] After few years in 1930, a combined recovery cum intensive care unit (ICU) in a surgical ward was established in Germany.[6] With these, the concept of building a separate area dedicated to monitor and manage more seriously ill came into place. Over the next 2–3 decades, almost all hospitals had such recovery or ICUs.[7] Two important events which are always remembered as they caused a major evolution in the field of critical care are Copenhagen's polio epidemic and the Second World War. Copenhagen polio epidemic during the 1950s affected a large number of people leading to respiratory failure.[2,5] Negative pressure mechanical ventilators (the iron lung) was used for respiratory support and saved many lives during that epidemic. During the Second World War, shock units were established by Dr Max Harry Weil and Dr Hebert Shubin for the recognition and treatment of critically ill patients.[2] These two events seem to define what would constitute care in the critical care unit.

Over the next few decades, the appearance of the ICU also evolved.[7] Initially, ICUs were usually located at isolated places and looked mysterious and frightening.[8] All personnel, including physicians, nursing staff, and visitors dressed in fully covered dresses with caps, masks, and gowns. All this used to give a very frightening look, making patients as well as visitors anxious. There was also an assumption that visitors who come to see these patients were a cause of increased anxiety, physiological stress, and increased the chances of infections.[9-12] Therefore, visiting hours were limited.[8,11]

Initially, for decades, ICU were primarily managed by anesthesiologists and internists and were recognized as medical or surgical ICU.[13] Later in the US, a concept of separate specialty ICU, such as respiratory, cardiac, and neurosurgical ICU, was introduced. Most of the ICUs were open and the patients admitted from different specialties were seen by their respective admitting physician, so that different patients admitted in that ICU were seen by different physicians. However, it was realized later that, irrespective of the specialty they came from, these critically ill patients had similar pathophysiological abnormalities. Further, the outcome of these patients was better when managed by a specialized critical care team—involving critical care physician, nurses, and physiotherapist—who were dedicated to the ICU as compared to being managed by the admitting physician.[14,15] Over a period, it was also realized that intensivist or critical care physicians had a significant role in improvement of the outcome of these patients and many hospitals in the West started special training for critical care physicians.

## ADVANCES IN VENTILATORS

The first ventilator, iron lung, was used in Haward Medical School in 1927 by Phillips Drinker and Shaw.[16,17] Later, this was modified by John Emerson. These machines used intermittent negative pressure around the body to create a negative pressure in the airways which was used to suck air inside.[17] For this, the person was kept in a chamber in such a way that whole body, except the head was in the chamber with an airtight collar around the neck. By applying a negative pressure in the chamber, the lung was expanded and ventilation achieved. Its use was very cumbersome. It was not suitable for totally paralytic patients. For such patients, Ibsen, a Danish anesthesiologist, suggested tracheostomy and manual ambu bag ventilation.[17,18] In 1947, piston ventilator was introduced by Mörch and later modified by Engsrom and Emerson.[19,20] These ventilators are usually referred as first generation ventilators.[21] These machines were used successfully for ventilation of even for totally paralyzed patients and revolutionized the care of patients with respiratory failure. However, these ventilators had only volume controlled mode and patient triggering was not possible. There was no or limited means to monitor patients on these ventilators. The second generation ventilators, which include Seimens servo and Ohio 560, incorporated monitoring of some parameters, such as tidal volume and respiratory rate.[21] Another important feature was that these ventilators could deliver patient triggered inspiration. These ventilators also incorporated basic alarms, such as high pressure, high rate, and low tidal volume. With these ventilators, initially intermittent mandatory ventilation (IMV) and later, synchronous IMV (SIMV) mode of ventilation came into use. Third generation ventilators were characterized by the presence of microprocessor control system. With the help of microprocessor, virtually any mode of gas delivery was possible. These ventilators are more responsive to patients demand and flow triggering became a reality.[21,22] All these ventilators can provide pressure support, pressure control, volume control, and SIMV mode of ventilation. SIMV was not only available in volume ventilation but also pressure ventilation and pressure support could be applied during the spontaneous breaths. These ventilators also provide extensive monitoring of patients as well as display almost all ventilatory parameters. These ventilators also give data in the form of waveforms of pressure, flow, and volume along with pressure-volume and flow-volume loops. Current ventilators, the so called fourth generation, are most advanced and complex. These are very versatile ventilators and may be used in any setting and can provide any mode.[21]

## THERAPEUTIC ADVANCES

Over the period, there has been tremendous advancement in the technological aspects in the field of critical care. For example, the initial ventilator which was large and cumbersome to use has been replaced with more advanced, small, easily portable, and easy to use newer ventilator.[21] There has been lots of research in the field of critical care during the last few years. However, there has been no significant addition to the therapeutics aspect. With this research, however, we were able to get rid many practices which were thought to be "standard of care" sometimes back. Most important among these was use of activated protein-C for management for septic shock, which till few years back was endorsed by many societies.[23] However, its usefulness was clearly refuted by later research.[24] Similarly, use of sedation and muscle relaxant was almost a universal practice with the assumption that it helps in better ventilation and reduces patient discomfort. Now, it has been well established that excessive use of sedation and paralytic agents is associated with a worse outcome.[25] Other practices, such as threshold for blood transfusion, albumin infusion, renal dose of dopamine, tight glycemic control, routine corticosteroid use for septic shock, and insertion of pulmonary catheter has also been almost stopped universally.[26-30]

One of the major therapeutic advancement that has occurred in the field of critical care is low tidal volume ventilation and the concept of permissive hypercapnia.[31] Low tidal volume ventilation strategy has significantly changed the outcome of patient with adult respiratory distress syndrome (ARDS) and now has been universally accepted as "standard of care".[32]

## ORGANIZATIONAL COLLABORATION

Over the years, it was recognized that there had been heterogeneity in the management of critically ill patients and a need for establishment of a scientific organization(s) was also felt. As a result, many organizations, such as The Society of Critical Care Medicine, The European Society of Intensive Care Medicine, and the World Federation of Societies of Intensive and Critical Care Medicine were established.[33-35] The objectives were to promote the awareness, foster research and education, provide recommendations, and collaboration among the intensive care physicians over the globe. With the establishment of these organizations, there has been a significant improvement and uniformity in various aspect in this filed, such as standard of ICU care, critical care delivery, management of various infections, insulin infusion, etc.[36-38] Surviving Sepsis Campaign (SSC) is another initiative which was started in 2002 with the goal to reduce mortality due to sepsis to 25%.[39] Subsequently, SSC came up with guidelines for management of sepsis, one of the common causes of critical illness.[39,40] These guidelines are updated periodically to incorporate new evidence in to practice.[32,41]

Another important development that has occurred due to the efforts of these organizations is the continued research in the field of critical care. There is now a better understanding of the pathophysiology of critical illness and various syndromes seen among these patients. Disease processes, such as sepsis, ARDS, ventilator induced pneumonia, are now defined more precisely.[40,42] Further, definitions and management of diseases are updated whenever new research suggests there is a need to do so.[42] With this, the heterogeneity in the diagnosis and management of critically ill patients has been minimized. Researchers have also come up with various scores which can predict the outcome and allow risk stratification of these critically ill patients. Among these Acute Physiology and Chronic Health Evaluation, Simplified Acute Physiology Score, and Sepsis-related Organ Failure Assessment scores are commonly used.[43-46]

Like many fields in medicine, critical care is also evolving. Newer data and technology is leading to an ever changing management strategy. Various protocols like early goal directed therapy for sepsis get constantly questioned and modified. Fundamentally, critical care revolves around supporting a seriously ill patient till the underlying disease recovers. Support mainly revolves around ventilatory, cardiac, and renal support. The prevention and management of infection that occurs with this supportive care is also important. Infection can itself be a cause of the illness requiring supportive care due to shock and multi-organ failure. For an intensivist, it is therefore important to understand basic respiratory and cardiac physiology so as to able to apply this support in the best possible manner. The basic principle of medicine "first do no harm" is all the more important in an ICU setting. Many ICU related complications kill the patients rather than the disease itself. It is, therefore, essential to weigh the risk versus benefit of many interventions we do in the ICU. The highest mortality in any hospital occurs in the ICU. It is to be expected as the sickest patients get admitted there. But many patients die due to ICU related care and complications. There is, therefore, a need for proper critical care training with regular updates so that the best available care can be provided to these very sick patients.

Intensive care unit is also expensive. A cost effective analysis is required for many of the interventions that are done in the ICU. Unfortunately, this is rarely done and the cost of ICU care with disposables and multiple interventions has sky rocketed. In developing countries, there is a need to develop and evaluate local less expensive ICU care methods. Many techniques, devices, and interventions in the ICU can be done in a much more cost effective manner without compromising on patient care.

As has already been discussed, ICU's have a high mortality. With an aging population, many terminally ill patients or patients with advanced neurocognitive disease will be admitted in the ICU. Firstly, one needs to evaluate the need for prolonged ICU care in such patients. Many could get a better quality support and care outside an ICU setting. Secondly, most critical care physicians are not trained in discussing end of life issues with patients or their relatives. This is an essential part of ICU care and needs to be addressed as a part of training in critical care.

Critical care has, therefore, evolved substantially both in technique and philosophy over the last few decades. Newer devices and evidence-based guidelines are helping in providing better care in the ICU and this has helped to decrease overall mortality. ICU care also needs a humane touch as this gets often forgotten with all the equipment and tubes around and in the patient.

## CONCLUSION

Critical care has evolved significantly over last few decades. In the evolution process, there has been tremendous contributions from eminent researchers and physicians across the globe. There is lots of heterogeneity in critical care services. Various scientific bodies have contributed in making the critical care universally homogeneous. However, there is still lots of scope for improvement. Critical care is still quite expensive and out of reach to many who need it. Future efforts are required to establish international collaboration for conducting more trials, making it more homogeneous and to bring down the cost of care to make it affordable to every body who need it.

> ## Editor's Comment
>
> *Critical care has an ancient history though it has evolved substantially both in technique and philosophy in the last century or so. Newer devices and evidence-based guidelines have helped to provide an improved care which has significantly decreased the overall mortality. There is an ever increasing number of intensive care unit (ICU) admissions with an aging population. Many terminally ill patients, including those with incurable and advanced neurocognitive disease, are now admitted for the ICU care. Most of such patients need prolonged ICU hospitalization with little benefit in the survival or quality of life. Several of them could get a better quality support and care outside an ICU setting. Critical care physicians need adequate sensitization and training in handling issues related to a humane approach in the care of terminally sick patients.*
>
> ***Surinder K Jindal***

## REFERENCES


1. Vincent JL, Singer M, Marini JJ, Moreno R, Levy M, Matthay MA, et al. Thirty years of critical care medicine. *Crit Care.* 2010;14(3):311.
2. Grenvik A, Pinsky MR. Evolution of the intensive care unit as a clinical center and critical care medicine as a discipline. *Crit Care Clin.* 2009;25(1):239-50, x.
3. Vincent JL. Critical care—where have we been and where are we going? *Crit Care.* 2013;17 Suppl 1:S2.
4. Munro CL. The "lady with the lamp" illuminates critical care today. *Am J Crit Care.* 2010;19(4):315-7.
5. Safar P, Dekornfeld TJ, Pearson JW, Redding JS. The intensive care unit. A three year experience at Baltimore city hospitals. *Anaesthesia.* 1961;16:275-84.
6. Hanson CW 3rd, Durbin CG Jr, Maccioli GA, Deutschman CS, Sladen RN, Pronovost PJ, et al. The anesthesiologist in critical care medicine: past, present, and future. *Anesthesiology.* 2001;95(3):781-8.
7. Hilberman M. The evolution of intensive care units. *Crit Care Med.* 1975;3(4):159-65.
8. Berwick DM, Kotagal M. Restricted visiting hours in ICUs: time to change. *JAMA.* 2004;292(6):736-7.
9. Berti D, Ferdinande P, Moons P. Beliefs and attitudes of intensive care nurses toward visits and open visiting policy. *Intensive Care Med.* 2007;33(6):1060-5.
10. Lee MD, Friedenberg AS, Mukpo DH, Conray K, Palmisciano A, Levy MM. Visiting hours policies in New England intensive care units: strategies for improvement. *Crit Care Med.* 2007;35(2):497-501.
11. Hunter JD, Goddard C, Rothwell M, Ketharaju S, Cooper H. A survey of intensive care unit visiting policies in the United Kingdom. *Anaesthesia.* 2010;65(11):1101-5.
12. Fumagalli S, Boncinelli L, Lo Nostro A, Valoti P, Baldereschi G, Di Bari M, et al. Reduced cardiocirculatory complications with unrestrictive visiting policy in an intensive care unit: results from a pilot, randomized trial. *Circulation.* 2006;113(7):946-52.
13. Pronovost PJ, Angus DC, Dorman T, Robinson KA, Dremsizov TT, Young TL. Physician staffing patterns and clinical outcomes in critically ill patients: a systematic review. *JAMA.* 2002;288(17):2151-62.
14. Carson SS, Stocking C, Podsadecki T, Christenson J, Pohlman A, MacRae S, et al. Effects of organizational change in the medical intensive care unit of a teaching hospital: a comparison of 'open' and 'closed' formats. *JAMA.* 1996;276(4):322-8.

15. Ghorra S, Reinert SE, Cioffi W, Buczko G, Simms HH. Analysis of the effect of conversion from open to closed surgical intensive care unit. *Ann Surg.* 1999;229(2):163-71.

16. Drinker P, Shaw LA. An apparatus for the prolonged administration of artificial respiration: I. A design for adults and children. *J Clin Invest.* 1929;7(2):229-47.

17. Ibsen B. The anaesthetist's viewpoint on the treatment of respiratory complications in poliomyelitis during the epidemic in Copenhagen, 1952. *Proc R Soc Med.* 1954;47(1):72-4.

18. Ibsen B. Treatment of respiratory complications in poliomyelitis; the anesthetist's viewpoint. *Dan Med Bull.* 1954;1(1):9-12.

19. Moerch ET. Controlled respiration by means of special automatic machines as used in Sweden and Denmark [Abstract]. *Proc R Soc Med.* 1947;40(10):603-7.

20. Bjork VO, Engstrom CG. The treatment of ventilatory insufficiency after pulmonary resection with tracheostomy and prolonged artificial ventilation. *J Thorac Surg.* 1955;30(3):356-67.

21. Kacmarek RM. The mechanical ventilator: past, present, and future. *Respir Care.* 2011;56(8):1170-80.

22. Williams P, Kratohvil J, Ritz R, Hess DR, Kacmarek RM. Pressure support and pressure assist/control: are there differences? An evaluation of the newest intensive care unit ventilators. *Respir Care.* 2000;45(10):1169-81.

23. Bernard GR, Vincent JL, Laterre PF, LaRosa SP, Dhainaut JF, Lopez-Rodriguez A, et al. Efficacy and safety of recombinant human activated protein C for severe sepsis. *N Engl J Med.* 2001;344(10):699-709.

24. Ranieri VM, Thompson BT, Barie PS, Dhainaut JF, Douglas IS, Finfer S, et al. Drotrecogin alfa (activated) in adults with septic shock. *N Engl J Med.* 2012;366(22):2055-64.

25. Girard TD, Kress JP, Fuchs BD, Thomason JW, Schweickert WD, Pun BT, et al. Efficacy and safety of a paired sedation and ventilator weaning protocol for mechanically ventilated patients in intensive care (Awakening and Breathing Controlled trial): a randomised controlled trial. *Lancet.* 2008;371(9607):126-34.

26. Bellomo R, Chapman M, Finfer S, Hickling K, Myburgh J. Low-dose dopamine in patients with early renal dysfunction: a placebo-controlled randomised trial. Australian and New Zealand Intensive Care Society (ANZICS) Clinical Trials Group. *Lancet.* 2000;356(9248):2139-43.

27. van den Berghe G, Wouters P, Weekers F, Verwaest C, Bruyninckx F, Schetz M, et al. Intensive insulin therapy in critically ill patients. *N Engl J Med.* 2001;345(19):1359-67.

28. Finfer S, Chittock DR, Su SY, Blair D, Foster D, Dhingra V, et al. Intensive versus conventional glucose control in critically ill patients. *N Engl J Med.* 2009;360(13):1283-97.

29. Sprung CL, Annane D, Keh D, Moreno R, Singer M, Freivogel K, et al. Hydrocortisone therapy for patients with septic shock. *N Engl J Med.* 2008;358(2):111-24.

30. Wheeler AP, Bernard GR, Thompson BT, Schoenfeld D, Wiedemann HP, deBoisblanc B, et al. Pulmonary-artery versus central venous catheter to guide treatment of acute lung injury. *N Engl J Med.* 2006;354(21):2213-24.

31. Ventilation with lower tidal volumes as compared with traditional tidal volumes for acute lung injury and the acute respiratory distress syndrome. The Acute Respiratory Distress Syndrome Network. *N Engl J Med.* 2000;342(18):1301-8.

32. Dellinger RP, Levy MM, Rhodes A, Annane D, Gerlach H, Opal SM, et al. Surviving Sepsis Campaign: international guidelines for management of severe sepsis and septic shock, 2012. *Intensive Care Med.* 2013;39(2):165-228.

33. Weil MH. The Society of Critical Care Medicine, its history and its destiny. *Crit Care Med.* 1973;1(1):1-4.

34. World Federation of Societies of Intensive and Critical Care Medicine. Available from: http://wwwworld-critical-careorg/indexphp?option=com_content&view=article&id=4&Itemid=4. [Accessed on 23 Aug 2015].

35. European Society of Intensive Care Medicine. Available from: http://wwwesicmorg/about. [Accessed on 23 Aug 2015].

36. Thompson DR, Hamilton DK, Cadenhead CD, Swoboda SM, Schwindel SM, Anderson DC, et al. Guidelines for intensive care unit design. *Crit Care Med.* 2012;40(5):1586-600.

37. Brilli RJ, Spevetz A, Branson RD, Campbell GM, Cohen H, Dasta JF, et al. Critical care delivery in the intensive care unit: defining clinical roles and the best practice model. *Crit Care Med.* 2001;29(10):2007-19.

38. Jacobi J, Bircher N, Krinsley J, Agus M, Braithwaite SS, Deutschman C, et al. Guidelines for the use of an insulin infusion for the management of hyperglycemia in critically ill patients. *Crit Care Med.* 2012;40(12):3251-76.

39. Dellinger RP, Carlet JM, Masur H, Gerlach H, Calandra T, Cohen J, et al. Surviving Sepsis Campaign guidelines for management of severe sepsis and septic shock. *Crit Care Med*. 2004;32(3):858-73.
40. Levy MM, Fink MP, Marshall JC, Abraham E, Angus D, Cook D, et al. 2001 SCCM/ESICM/ACCP/ATS/SIS International Sepsis Definitions Conference. *Crit Care Med*. 2003;31(4):1250-6.
41. Dellinger RP, Levy MM, Carlet JM, Bion J, Parker MM, Jaeschke R, et al. Surviving Sepsis Campaign: international guidelines for management of severe sepsis and septic shock: 2008. *Intensive Care Med*. 2008;34(1):17-60.
42. Ranieri VM, Rubenfeld GD, Thompson BT, Ferguson ND, Caldwell E, Fan E, et al. Acute respiratory distress syndrome: the Berlin Definition. *JAMA*. 2012;307(23):2526-33.
43. Knaus WA, Draper EA, Wagner DP, Zimmerman JE. APACHE II: a severity of disease classification system. *Crit Care Med*. 1985;13(10):818-29.
44. Le Gall JR, Lemeshow S, Saulnier F. A new Simplified Acute Physiology Score (SAPS II) based on a European/North American multicenter study. *JAMA*. 1993;270(24):2957-63.
45. Vincent JL, Moreno R, Takala J, Willatts S, De Mendonca A, Bruining H, et al. The SOFA (Sepsis-related Organ Failure Assessment) score to describe organ dysfunction/failure. On behalf of the Working Group on Sepsis-Related Problems of the European Society of Intensive Care Medicine. *Intensive Care Med*. 1996;22(7):707-10.
46. Howell MD, Talmor D, Schuetz P, Hunziker S, Jones AE, Shapiro NI. Proof of principle: the predisposition, infection, response, organ failure sepsis staging system. *Crit Care Med*. 2011;39(2):322-7.

World Clin Pulm Crit Care Med. 2016;4(1):10-35.

# Assisted Ventilation

***Ritesh Agarwal** MD DM, **Inderpaul S Sehgal** MD DNB DM,
**Sahajal Dhooria** MD DM, **Ashutosh N Aggarwal** MD DM

Department of Pulmonary Medicine, Postgraduate Institute of Medical Education and Research
Chandigarh, India

## *ABSTRACT*

Mechanical ventilation is an integral and important component of critical care. The management of a mechanically ventilated patient requires a concerted effort of a multidisciplinary team of clinicians, nurses, respiratory therapists, and others to optimize therapeutic outcomes. The last three decades have enhanced our understanding of mechanical ventilation with the knowledge that the ventilator itself can cause significant injury to the lung parenchyma. This has led to a paradigm shift in setting of the ventilator with adoption of lower tidal volumes. All physicians involved in management of critically ill patients, directly or indirectly should be able to understand the basic principles of the functioning of a mechanical ventilator. The aim of this article is to help clinicians and nonclinicians understand the concepts of mechanical ventilation and apply this knowledge in optimizing the care of their patients.

## INTRODUCTION

Mechanical ventilation is the provision of assisted ventilation to patients with acute or chronic respiratory failure. It is a life-saving procedure in the management of patients with failing cardiorespiratory function. In fact, the advent of assisted ventilation is responsible for the continued growth of the specialty of critical care. It was in the 16th century that Vesalius proposed the concept of assisted ventilation.[1] In the 18th century, ventilation by mechanical bellows was attempted in Europe. Around the middle of 19th century, devices that applied subambient pressure outside the body were introduced. These negative

---

*Corresponding author
Email: agarwal.ritesh@outlook.in

pressure ventilators were put to extensive clinical use during the polio epidemic. However, it is the 20th century that has really seen the exponential growth of mechanical ventilation.[1,2] In the last five decades, mechanical ventilators have not only changed enormously in appearance (from bulky to compact devices), but have also become more sophisticated and versatile. Current generations of ventilators have enhanced microprocessor chips that control flow and pressure intelligently for optimal ventilation of the critically ill patient. The intensive care unit (ICU) structure has changed significantly with several ICUs being open in nature.[3] This warrants that the treating physician himself can understand the condition of the patient with regards to the ventilation and also comprehend the basic ventilatory settings. Further, a knowledge of basic concepts of ventilation will sharpen the treatment acumen of the involved physicians. Ventilatory support can be delivered either by invasive methods (endotracheal tube or tracheostomy) or by noninvasively (oronasal mask, facial mask). Noninvasive ventilation (NIV) has the advantage of avoiding artificial airways and their attendant complications [laryngeal injury, tracheal stenosis, ventilator-associated pneumonia (VAP), and others]. Further, the patient is able to communicate, take feeds orally, and does not require sedation. The use of NIV is also associated with shorter hospital and ICU stay, avoids the need of intubation, and reduced mortality especially in respiratory failure due to chronic obstructive pulmonary disease (COPD) and heart failure.[4-9] In this article, we provide a basic overview on the current concepts associated with invasive mechanical ventilation.

## OBJECTIVES

The purpose of mechanical ventilation is to provide assisted ventilation to a patient with respiratory failure. The following are the objectives of mechanical ventilation: (i) improve alveolar ventilation by increasing the respiratory rate (fR) and tidal volume (VT), and thus the minute ventilation. This is applicable to any patient who presents with neuromuscular respiratory failure such as myasthenia gravis, Guillain-Barré syndrome, snake envenoming and others; (ii) improve arterial oxygenation by improving gas exchange by opening the collapsed alveoli; and (iii) reduce the work of breathing by unloading the respiratory muscles by driving gas into the lungs under positive pressure.

The aforementioned benefits of mechanical ventilation are useful for reversing life-threatening hypoxemia, correcting respiratory acidosis, preventing atelectasis, reversing respiratory muscle fatigue, permitting sedation and/or neuromuscular blockade for operative anesthesia and others, decreasing the systemic oxygen consumption, and myriad of other benefits.[10]

Mechanical ventilation is indicated in any patient with respiratory failure severe enough to cause organ dysfunction or threat to life itself. In practice, respiratory

| Table 1: Common Indications for Assisted Ventilation in Day-to-day Practice | |
|---|---|
| **Type 1** | **Type 2** |
| • Acute respiratory distress syndrome<br>• Acute pulmonary edema<br>• Pneumonia<br>• Severe acute asthma | • Acute exacerbations of chronic obstructive pulmonary disease<br>• Guillain-Barré syndrome<br>• Myasthenia gravis |

| Table 2: Clinical and Laboratory Indicators of Inadequate Ventilation | | |
|---|---|---|
| | **Normal** | **Indicators for assisted ventilation** |
| **Ventilation** | | |
| Respiratory rate (per minute) | 12–20 | <10 or >35 |
| Tidal volume (mL/kg) | 6–8 | <5 |
| Vital capacity (mL/kg) | 65–75 | <10 |
| Negative inspiratory pressure (cm $H_2O$) | 75–100 | <20 |
| Minute ventilation (L/minute) | 5–6 | >10 or <4 |
| $PaCO_2$ (mmHg) | 35–45 | >55* |
| Dead space to tidal volume ratio | 0.25–0.40 | >0.60 |
| **Oxygenation** | | |
| $PaO_2$ (mmHg) | 70–100 | <55 |
| Alveolar-arterial gradient (mmHg) | 25–65 | >450** |

*Except in patients with chronic hypercapnia.
**On 100% oxygen supplementation.

failure is said to be present if the arterial partial pressure of oxygen ($PaO_2$) value is less than 60 mmHg while breathing room air. Respiratory failure is classified as type 1 (or hypoxemic respiratory failure) if the arterial partial pressure of carbon dioxide ($PaCO_2$) level is less than 45 mmHg or type 2 (or hypercapnic respiratory failure) if the $PaCO_2$ level is more than or equal to 45 mmHg.[11] Assisted ventilation is however not required in all patients with respiratory failure but only in those who worsen despite optimal medical therapy and oxygen supplementation.[12] The common indications for mechanical ventilation are shown in table 1. Several parameters based on vital signs, pulmonary function tests, and arterial blood gas analysis can assist clinicians in deciding when to initiate mechanical ventilation (Table 2).

## BASIC TERMINOLOGIES OF MECHANICAL VENTILATION

Almost all mechanical ventilators used currently are positive pressure ventilators that force gas to move from high pressure (ventilator) to low pressure (lungs)

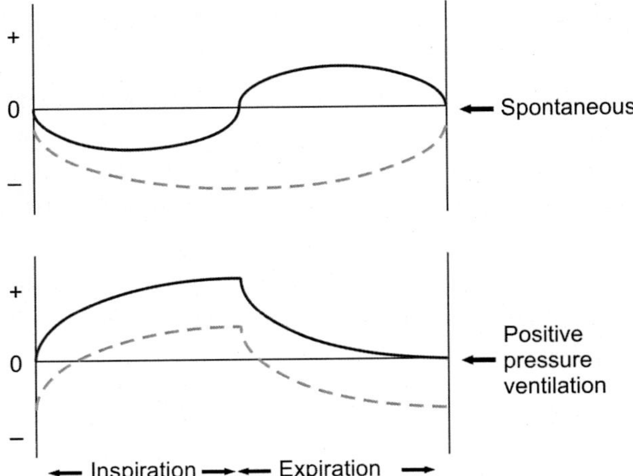


**Figure 1:** Alveolar pressure (solid curve) and intrapleural pressure (dotted curve) in a spontaneously breathing patient and during positive pressure ventilation.

due to application of positive pressure. Negative pressure ventilators are rarely used in critical care. The thoracic pressure variations during positive pressure ventilation are the opposite of that seen during spontaneous breathing such that during inspiration the intrathoracic pressure increases while it decreases during expiration. Due to positive pressure, the alveolar pressure builds progressively and becomes more positive during inspiration. This positive pressure is transmitted to the visceral pleura and the intrapleural pressure also becomes positive during inspiration (Figure 1). At the end of inspiration, the ventilator stops delivering positive pressure. Thus, the pressure in the proximal airway falls to zero but the alveolar pressure is still positive. This gradient leads to passive exhalation. It is important to understand certain commonly used terms in the setting of mechanical ventilators to understand their functioning.

*Trigger*: This term is defined as the signal that opens the inspiratory valve and initiates the inspiratory cycle by allowing pressurized gas to enter the lungs of the patient.

*Cycle*: This is the signal that stops the inspiratory cycle and opens the expiratory valve allowing initiation of exhalation. Cycling can be triggered by preset volume or flow (i.e., once the VT goal or preset decline in flow is reached), pressure (once the pressure limit is achieved), or time (duration of inspiratory cycle).

*Limit*: This is the threshold that controls gas flow into the lungs, and is different from the cycling variable. Technically, cycling (or alarm setting) opens the expiratory valve while limit maintains the gas flow without opening the exhalation valve.

*Tidal volume*: Tidal volume is the amount of gas that enters and leaves the lung with each respiratory cycle. Traditionally, the recommended VT has been about 10 mL/kg. However, in the landmark Acute Respiratory Distres Syndrome Network (ARDS Net) trial, it was shown that a VT of 6 mL/kg improves survival in patients with acute respiratory distress syndrome (ARDS).[13] Although patients without ARDS are still ventilated with large VTs (about 8–10 mL/kg), recent studies have shown that use of higher VTs can cause ventilator-associated lung injury (VALI) even in patients with normal lungs.[14-22] Recognition of this fact has led to a paradigm shift in the ventilatory management with use of lower VTs even in those without ARDS.[23,24]

*Respiratory rate*: In patients with normal lungs, the fR is generally maintained at 14–18 breaths/minute. In those with obstructive lung physiology, the fR is set at 8–12 breaths/minute; this increases the expiratory time and allows exhalation of as much air as possible. In restrictive lung physiology, higher fRs are easily tolerated. In general, the fR and VT can be easily manipulated depending on the patient's arterial blood gases.

*Fraction of inspired oxygen*: The fraction of inspired oxygen ($FiO_2$) is delivered along with the pressurized gas. The modern ventilators have oxygen blenders that blend the desired amount of oxygen with air to deliver the precise amount of oxygen. It has been long recognized that $FiO_2$ greater than 0.6 is potentially toxic and can induce oxygen toxicity if given for prolonged periods. Hence, it is important to minimize oxygen toxicity by maintaining the lowest $FiO_2$ that achieves oxygen saturation ($SpO_2$) of 90% corresponding to $PaO_2$ of approximately 60 mmHg.[25]

*Positive end-expiratory pressure*: In the normal lungs, the intrathoracic pressure at the end of exhalation approaches that of atmospheric pressure. The intrapleural pressure is slightly negative and this maintains a resting volume of air inside the lungs, which is known as functional residual capacity. In the modern ventilators, the end-expiratory pressure can be maintained above the atmospheric pressure and is termed as positive end-expiratory pressure (PEEP). PEEP plays an important role in maintaining alveolar patency, which is reduced during mechanical ventilation due to surfactant loss and alveolar instability leading to alveolar collapse. Continuous positive airway pressure (CPAP) is technically the same as PEEP; however, the term CPAP is employed in patients who are breathing spontaneously.[26] The PEEP that is applied is also referred to as extrinsic PEEP or applied PEEP to differentiate from intrinsic PEEP or auto-PEEP, which results from incomplete emptying of alveolar gas at the end of exhalation thereby elevating the alveolar pressure relative to airway opening (mouth) pressure.[27]

In patients with expiratory flow limitation (e.g., COPD) or increased airflow resistance (e.g., narrow endotracheal tube, high minute ventilation), air trapping at end-expiration worsens with each successive breath, leading to an increase in alveolar pressures and functional residual capacity, termed as dynamic hyperinflation.[28] Auto-PEEP can also occur without dynamic hyperinflation if there is active contraction of expiratory muscles during expiration. Auto-PEEP can be measured by occluding the expiratory limb of the patient circuit and delaying the delivery of the next breath.[29]

Both PEEP and auto-PEEP can reduce venous return and cardiac output by direct transmission of positive alveolar pressure to the intrapleural space. PEEP (and auto-PEEP) can also lead to barotrauma. Auto-PEEP can increase the inspiratory work of breathing as the patient needs to generate a larger effort to overcome the auto-PEEP before reaching the pressure level to trigger the ventilator.

*Peak inspiratory flow*: The movement of gas inside the lung is a measure of the rate of airflow multiplied by time. The higher the peak inspiratory flow the shorter the inspiratory cycle and vice versa. During mechanical ventilation, the inspiratory flow rate is usually set at 60 L/minute. However, in patients with obstructive lung disease, a higher peak flows can technically decrease the inspiratory time and in turn allow a prolonged expiratory time thus helping in better emptying of the lungs.[30] An inappropriately low inspiratory flow relative to the patient's demand can increase the work of breathing as it leads to generation of high negative intrapleural pressures due to the patient perception that the ventilatory requirement is unlikely to be met at the set inspiratory flow.

*Sighs*: Most ventilators are capable of providing periodic large volume breaths termed as "sighs". When sighs are used, they are usually set at 1.5–2 times the VT and delivered every 2–3 minutes, mimicking the sighing frequency of a normal individual.[31] The rationale for the use of sighs is that periodic hyperinflation is likely to decrease the risk of atelectasis. Whether they are useful in patients already receiving PEEP or larger VT is not known. Further, sighs should be avoided if they are associated with high ventilating pressures, particularly in patients with ARDS receiving PEEP.

*Peak pressure*: Pressure measurements in a ventilated patient reflect the proximal airway pressures. Peak pressure (Ppeak) is the peak inspiratory pressure that is measured at the end of the inspiratory cycle. The pressure then falls back to baseline unless PEEP has been applied (Figure 1). A high Ppeak represents either increased alveolar pressure, lung hyperinflation, or airway resistance (Raw). In general, the Ppeak is usually maintained below 35–40 cm $H_2O$ to limit lung damage.

*Plateau pressure*: This is the pressure measured at the end of an inspiratory cycle with an inspiratory hold, i.e., with the inspiratory valve closed (Figure 2). This results in static conditions with no flow, representing the pressure in the alveoli. An increase in Ppeak without a proportionate increase in plateau pressure (Pplat)

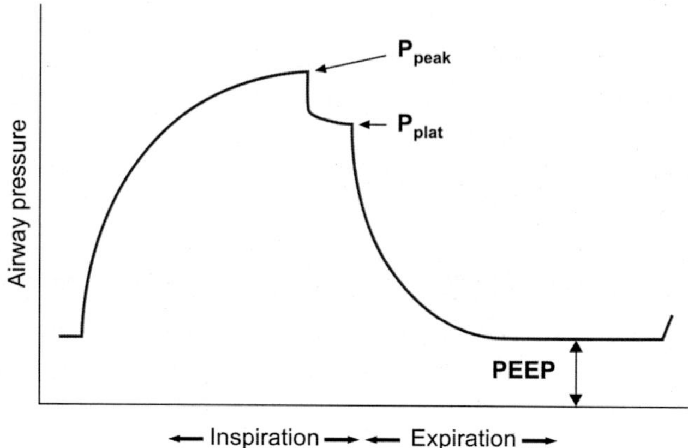



**Figure 2:** Airway pressure recording during a mechanically delivered breath. An end-inspiratory pause produces a rapid decline from peak pressure (Ppeak) to plateau pressure (Pplat). Exhalation then commences, and airway pressure drops gradually to baseline [or positive end-expiratory pressure (PEEP), in this example].

(Ppeak minus Pplat ≥10–15 cm $H_2O$) signifies airflow obstruction. A Pplat value less than 30 cm $H_2O$ is usually maintained to minimize VALI. The difference between Ppeak and Pplat is termed transairway pressure, and represents the pressure lost to Raw.

*Mean airway pressure*: This is the area enclosed by the airway pressure tracing for one complete respiratory cycle, divided by the duration of that cycle. It reflects the importance of both the amount and duration of pressure, and is the average pressure throughout the respiratory cycle. The mean airway pressure (MAP) has the maximum influence on oxygenation. It is calculated as [Ppeak × Inspiratory time (%) + PEEP × Expiratory time (%)]. A high MAP is associated with decrease in the cardiac output and pulmonary hypoperfusion while an MAP greater than 12 cm $H_2O$ contributes to barotrauma.[32,33]

*Lung compliance*: Compliance is defined as change in volume per unit change in pressure.[34] In a ventilated patient, the respiratory system (i.e., lungs and chest wall) has both a dynamic compliance (Cdyn) and a static compliance (Cstat). Static compliance is calculated by dividing the exhaled VT by Pplat (minus the PEEP),[11] i.e., Cstat = VT/(Pplat – PEEP). The normal Cstat in a ventilated patient is around 100 mL/cm $H_2O$. At values less than 25 mL/cm $H_2O$, the work of breathing is very high. A change in Cstat usually reflects a change in the elastic recoil of the lung parenchyma and conditions such as ARDS, air trapping, pulmonary edema, atelectasis, pneumonia, pneumothorax, or pleural effusion will all lower Cstat. Other conditions such as flail chest, pneumomediastinum, and abdominal distention can also lead to a similar change as Cstat also reflects compliance of the chest wall. The volume delivered by the ventilator divided by the Ppeak (minus the PEEP, if any), is the Cdyn,[12] i.e., Cdyn = VT/(Ppeak – PEEP). The Cdyn as with Cstat represents not only the compliance of the lungs and chest wall, but also the resistance of ventilator circuit and airways. Cdyn therefore decreases whenever Cstat falls or Raw increases.

Currently, it is possible to partition the static lung compliance (CL) into CL and chest wall compliance (Ccw) by measuring the esophageal pressure (Pes).[35] The Pes, which is a surrogate for pleural pressure (Ppl) is measured by placing an esophageal catheter (with a pressure transducer) in the lower one-third of the esophagus. The Cstat of the entire respiratory system ($Cstat_{RS}$) is calculated by dividing the VT by end-inspiratory pressure (subtracting the end-expiratory pressure), i.e., $Cstat_{RS}$ = Exhaled VT/(Pplat – PEEP). The Ccw ($Cstat_{cw}$) is measured by dividing the VT by end-inspiratory Pes (subtracting the end-expiratory Pes), i.e., $Cstat_{cw}$ = Exhaled VT/($Pes_{insp}$ – $Pes_{exp}$). The Cstat of the lung alone ($Cstat_{lung}$) is calculated by subtracting $Cstat_{cw}$ from $Cstat_{RS}$, i.e., $Cstat_{lung}$ = $Cstat_{RS}$ – $Cstat_{cw}$.

The Pes also provides another useful measurement, namely, the transpulmonary pressure (Ptp). The Ptp is the actual driving pressure for gas flow in the lung and is calculated as the difference between the alveolar pressure and the intrapleural pressure in the lungs, i.e., Ptp plat = Pplat – Pesinsp. The Ptp is the most important determinant of lung injury. It has been shown that the Ppl is relatively high and unpredictable in patients with ARDS,[36] and underscore the need for calculating the Ptp in ventilating difficult patients with ARDS. It is currently possible to perform continuous real-time Ptp monitoring with the newer ventilator Avea (CareFusion Technologies, Available from http://www.carefusion.com/medical-products/respiratory/ventilation/avea/). The Avea ventilator provides Ptp both during inspiration and expiration termed as Ptp plat and Ptp PEEP, respectively.

*Airway resistance*: The total resistance of the respiratory system is a sum of the Raw and tissue resistance, the former being the major contributor (about 80% to the total value).[37] The Raw is the driving pressure necessary to produce a given rate of airflow into the lungs. This driving pressure in the ventilated patient is approximated by the difference between Ppeak and Pplat. Flow corresponding to Ppeak is measured at the end of inspiration. Therefore, Raw = (Ppeak – Pplat)/flow. The normal Raw is less than 2.5 cm $H_2O$/L/second. With an artificial airway, this can increase to 6 cm $H_2O$/L/second or more, and may be even higher in patients with obstructive lung disease or airway secretions.

The changes in compliance and/or resistance are not uniformly distributed in a diseased lung, and thus different lung segments fill and empty at different rates. A low compliance (stiff) segment fills rapidly, but with a much smaller volume for the same filling pressure. A segment with high resistance fills slowly, but can accommodate normal volume if given sufficient time. The amount and rate of filling (and emptying) can be defined by a mathematical expression termed the "time constant".[38] Time constant is a product of compliance and resistance. One time constant allows 63% of either inspiratory or expiratory phase to occur. Three time constants allow about 95% of either phase, and five time constants theoretically allow nearly all of inspiration or expiration.

## CLASSIFICATION OF MECHANICAL VENTILATORS

Mechanical ventilators have been classified broadly depending on the control variable.[39-42] A "control variable" is the one that the ventilator manipulates to produce inspiration; it remains constant despite changes in the patient's pulmonary mechanics. For the beginner, it is only essential to remember that the common control variables are pressure, volume, and dual control. If the Ppeak remains constant as the load on the ventilator is varied, then the control variable is pressure. If the Ppeak changes with the change in the load but the VT remains constant, then the control variable is volume. Pressure and volume are interrelated, so only one of these (but not both) can be predetermined at a point in time (the independent variable) and the other becomes the dependent variable. However, the ventilator may switch from one control variable to the other either during a single inspiration (termed as dual control within a breath) or between breaths (termed as dual control, breath to breath). For each control variable, there are a limited number of inspiratory flow waveforms, which can be grouped into four basic categories: (i) rectangular (or square), (ii) descending ramp, (iii) sinusoidal and (iv) exponential.

## TRADITIONAL MODES OF MECHANICAL VENTILATION

*Control mode ventilation*: This is a time-triggered and volume- or time-cycled mode. It is currently employed only for apneic patients secondary to central nervous system depression, drug-induced sedation, or neuromuscular paralysis. The advantage of this mode is that a preset level of ventilation is always guaranteed. However, control mode ventilation (CMV) delivers a preselected rate, VT, and flow, independent of the patient's own respiratory efforts, without allowing any spontaneous breaths in between. Hence, it is poorly tolerated by awake patients or patients breathing spontaneously.

*Assist/control mode ventilation*: This is patient- or time-triggered and volume-cycled. An inspiratory cycle is initiated either by the patient's inspiratory effort or if no patient effort is detected within a specified time period, by a time signal within the ventilator (Figure 3). Every breath, whether patient-triggered or ventilator-triggered is fully supported by the ventilator and delivered at user-predefined

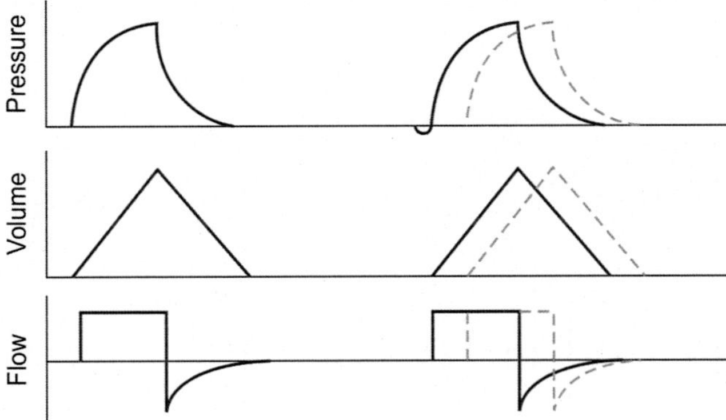

**Figure 3:** Airway pressure, lung volume and flow curves in relation to time during assist control mode of ventilation. The first breath is mandatory. The second breath is patient-triggered and occurs before the set time (dotted curve). This assisted breath delivers the same volume of gas at the same flow as the mandatory breath.

parameters. Thus, the ventilatory rate is determined either by the patient or by the specified rate, whichever is of higher frequency. Assist/control mode ventilation (ACMV) therefore allows the patient to increase his minute ventilation with minimum effort and at minimal metabolic cost by simply increasing the frequency of respiratory efforts. However, ACMV can lead to significant respiratory alkalosis in tachypneic patients. At high rates, this mode entails the risk of air trapping even in patients without airway obstruction, and thus patients frequently need to be sedated to optimize ventilation. Although in the older ventilators, (A) CMV meant volume cycling only, the newer ventilators have pressure-controlled continuous mandatory ventilation (PC-CMV), pressure-controlled synchronized intermittent mandatory ventilation (PC-SIMV) and others.

*Intermittent mandatory ventilation*: This delivers breaths at an operator-specified frequency, but differs from CMV in allowing unrestricted, unassisted spontaneous breathing between mechanical cycles. Synchronized intermittent mandatory ventilation (SIMV) allows these predetermined breaths to be delivered in concert with the patient's own efforts (Figure 4), and differs from ACMV in that only a preset number of breaths are assisted by the ventilator. Both these methods allow for a variation in the level of ventilatory support from near-total support to spontaneous breathing. Thus, patient can perform a variable amount of work with an added benefit of preset mandatory level of ventilation. Although considered as a good mode for both ventilating and weaning patients, this mode has been associated with the poorest outcome in terms of weaning.[43] Not all of patient's breaths are assisted and the spontaneous inspiratory work may be sufficiently high to preclude effective spontaneous breathing.[44,45] SIMV can also be combined with

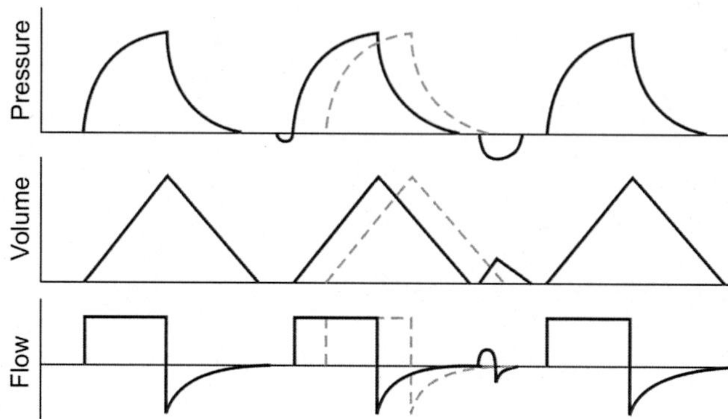

**Figure 4:** Airway pressure, lung volume and flow curves in relation to time during synchronized intermittent mandatory ventilation. The first breath is mandatory. The second breath is patient-triggered in the interval and one can observe that the ventilator is programmed to synchronize it with the patient's inspiratory effort. The third breath is initiated before the preset synchronization window and is therefore not assisted by the ventilator. The last breath is delivered as a mandatory breath when the patient fails to trigger another breath within the next synchronization window.

pressure support ventilation (PSV), where the spontaneous breaths are assisted by PS. However, even this mode is inferior as the respiratory center and respiratory muscles have to alter their output in anticipation of the next breath, which may either be mandatory or spontaneous.[31,44-47]

*Pressure support ventilation*: This is patient-triggered, flow-cycled, and pressure-limited (Figure 5). At the onset of inspiration, the pressure rises rapidly to an operator-specified value and is maintained at that level throughout inspiration. Inspiration is terminated when inspiratory airflow decelerates below a certain level during the terminal portion of inspiration. This low threshold is usually around 25% of the initial flow, although this can be adjusted by the clinician. When the pressure support level is chosen appropriately (judged by fR <30 breaths/minute and $SpO_2$ >90%), this mode is generally comfortable for most spontaneously breathing patients.[48] PSV reduces the work of breathing roughly in proportion to the pressure delivered. Additionally, lower levels can be used to overcome additional work of breathing imposed by artificial airways and ventilator circuits.[49] The pressure support required to overcome artificial Raw is however not adequate, generally being higher at low flow rates and lower at high flow rates. To overcome this, the newer ventilators have incorporated an additional mode called automatic tube compensation (ATC), which calculates the resistance across the endotracheal tube, and changes the pressure support accordingly.[50] PSV can also be used in combination with SIMV to support spontaneous breaths not assisted by the ventilator. The inherent disadvantage of PSV is that the VT depends on the level

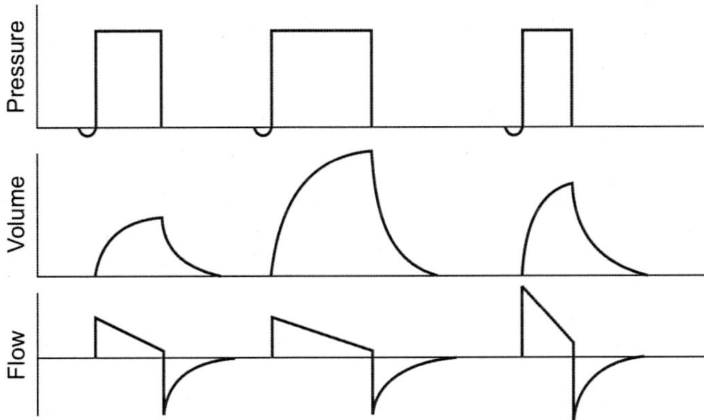


**Figure 5:** Airway pressure, lung volume and flow curves in relation to time during pressure support ventilation. When a breath is triggered, airway pressure rises and is maintained at the set level, with flow and tidal volume depending on the set pressure, respiratory system mechanics and patient effort. The first breath represents a situation (for comparison) where the patient triggers a breath and then remains fully passive. In the middle breath, the patient makes a small but prolonged inspiratory effort, resulting in a longer inspiratory time and a larger tidal volume. The last breath is more powerful, but brief, shortening the inspiratory time, but still generating a larger tidal volume than that during the passive breath.

of pressure support, impedance of the respiratory system, cycling frequency, and patient-ventilator synchrony. However, it is a useful modality both for delivering assisted ventilation at different levels of support as well as for gradual withdrawal of ventilatory support.[51]

*Pressure control ventilation*: This is time-triggered, time-cycled, and pressure-limited mode of ventilation. During inspiratory phase, a preset pressure is delivered, and this pressure remains at the operator-specified level throughout the inspiration (Figure 6). Like PSV, VT and inspiratory flow are dependent variables. However, unlike PSV, inspiration is terminated after a user-defined time period. The current ventilators offer pressure control ventilation (PCV) in the ACMV or SIMV modes, and are better tolerated than volume-controlled modes in some patients due to high flow rates. PCV is generally preferred in patients having persistently high airway pressures or those with documented barotrauma during volume-controlled ventilation.

*Continuous positive airway pressure*: This mode provides CPAP at operator-specified level throughout the ventilatory cycle; all breaths are spontaneous. CPAP thus offers the benefits of PEEP to spontaneously breathing patients. It improves oxygenation by recruiting collapsed alveoli and helps to reduce work of breathing in patients with dynamic hyperinflation and auto-PEEP. However, hyperinflation

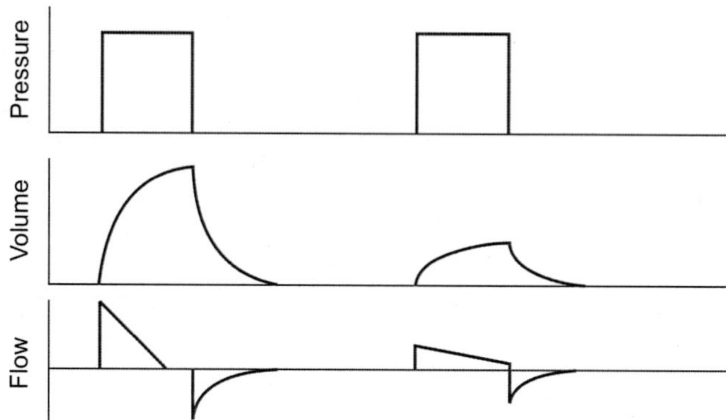



**Figure 6:** Airway pressure, lung volume, and flow curves in relation to time during pressure control ventilation in a paralyzed patient. The first tracing shows flow and tidal volume in a patient with normal lung mechanics. Lung compliance is decreased in the second tracing. At the same airway pressure, inspiratory flow is reduced and the expected tidal volume is not reached even until the termination of inspiration.

and work of breathing may increase if excessive levels of CPAP are used. CPAP is generally combined with PSV for weaning patients off mechanical ventilation.

## ADVANCED MODES OF MECHANICAL VENTILATION

The advances in technology over the last three decades have resulted in an "explosion" of different modes of mechanical ventilation, and every ventilator firm has a proprietary mode. In fact, it has become difficult even for the expert to keep abreast with the developments in the field. The examples of these newer modes of ventilation include: airway pressure release ventilation (bilevel ventilation, biphasic positive airway pressure, DuoPAP, Bi-level, Bi-vent), pressure-regulated volume control, adaptive support ventilation, proportional assist ventilation, volume-assured pressure support and others. Unfortunately, none of the newer modes of ventilation have been conclusively shown to be better than traditional modes of ventilation.

Many of these modes of ventilation are in fact "closed-loop control" wherein the ventilator employs the use of a feedback signal to adjust its output. As mentioned previously, only one variable (i.e., pressure or volume) can be independent at any moment, but the newer ventilators can switch between the two during a single inspiration, the so-called dual-control within a breath. The ventilator starts inspiration in volume control and then switch to pressure control or vice versa, if one or more preset thresholds are met (e.g., pressure control assist control with machine volume in the Avea ventilator).

Recently, a different classification has been proposed wherein the word targeting is used instead of control and is further divided into manual (set-point and dual), servo (simple and advanced), and automatic (adaptive, optimal and intelligent).[52] Although extremely intuitive, this classification is difficult to be understood by a beginner and is better left for experts.

## NONINVASIVE MECHANICAL VENTILATION

Noninvasive ventilation is the provision of ventilatory support to the lungs without the use of an artificial airway. The advent of NIV has revolutionized the treatment of diverse forms of acute respiratory failure (ARF). NIV not only reduces the need for invasive mechanical ventilation and its associated complications, but also reduces the complications associated with stay in the ICU, length of hospital stay, and mortality in patients with acute exacerbations of COPD and cardiogenic pulmonary edema.[6,53]

The term NIV encompasses a range of modes to augment alveolar ventilation without an artificial airway with CPAP and noninvasive positive pressure ventilation (NIPPV) being the most commonly used modes. In NIPPV, two different pressures are used, viz., inspiratory positive airway pressure (IPAP) and expiratory positive airway pressure (EPAP), whereas CPAP maintains a constant positive airway pressure throughout the respiratory cycle. Theoretically, NIPPV may confer an advantage over CPAP by reducing the work of breathing during inspiration by providing additional inspiratory pressure.[6] The best indications for the use of NIV include acute exacerbations of COPD and cardiogenic pulmonary edema that fails to respond to optimal medical therapy. NIV should be use judiciously in other situations such as pneumonia, ARDS, and severe acute asthma.[4,5,9,54-56] The contraindications to the use of NIV include altered mental status, hemodynamic instability, poor cough reflex, bulbar dysfunction and others.

In the critically ill patients, the use of critical care ventilator with oxygen blender is preferred over domiciliary ventilator with external oxygen supply for delivering NIV. As most patients with ARF are mouth breathers, an oronasal mask is preferred. In our ICU, we start with an IPAP/EPAP of 8/4 cm $H_2O$. IPAP is then increased in increments of 2–3 cm $H_2O$ (maximum 20 cm $H_2O$) to obtain an exhaled VT of 6 mL/kg and an fR of 30 breaths/minute. EPAP is increased in increments of 1–2 cm $H_2O$ (maximum 10 cm $H_2O$) to ensure an $SpO_2$ of 92% with the lowest $FiO_2$ possible. Generally, a trial of NIPPV is given for 1–4 hours while closely monitoring respiratory, cardiovascular, and arterial blood gas parameters. Importantly, facilities for intubation and invasive ventilation should be readily available for patients not improving or worsening with the use of NIV.

## PRACTICAL APPROACH TO INVASIVE MECHANICAL VENTILATION

Patients who fail treatment with oxygen and NIV generally require endotracheal intubation and invasive ventilation. The aim of invasive ventilation is to correct hypoxemia and maintain alveolar ventilation appropriate to patient's metabolic requirements. It has been recognized since 1970 that mechanical ventilation if not applied properly could cause harm.[57] A new era of ventilatory management began in 1990 when it was shown that prevention of pulmonary overdistension and permissive hypercapnia decreased mortality in patients with ARDS.[13,58] Although patients without acute lung injury (ALI) are still ventilated with large VTs, recent studies have shown that use of higher VTs can cause VALI even in patients with normal lungs. The current ventilatory strategy aims at minimizing complications of mechanical ventilation. The principles are to prevent additional alveolar injury and facilitate healing of the underlying condition. The ventilation is thus pressure-targeted employing lower VTs. The aim is to have blood gases within an acceptable physiological range and not complete normalization of physiological parameters (Table 3).

An important consideration is the ventilator or the mode that should be used for mechanically ventilating these patients. The choice of ventilator depends

**Table 3: Protocol for Ventilation in Different Categories of Respiratory Failure Employed at the Authors' Institute**

| | Restricted lung | Obstructed lung | Normal lung |
|---|---|---|---|
| Prototype | Acute respiratory distress syndrome | Severe acute asthma | Neuromuscular respiratory failure |
| Mode | V-ACMV | V-ACMV | V-ACMV |
| Initial tidal volumes | 4–6 mL/kg | 4–6 mL/kg | 6–8 mL/kg |
| Respiratory rate | 18–35/minute | 8–12/minute | 14–18/minute |
| PEEP | Based on $FiO_2$; 0.XX ($FiO_2$) × 20* | 5–8 cm $H_2O$ | Up to 5 cm $H_2O$ |
| Peak inspiratory flow | 40–60 L/minute | 80–100 L/minute | 60 L/minute |
| I:E | 1:1–1:2 | 1:3–1:6 | 1:2–1:3 |
| Flow waveform | Descending ramp | Square waveform | – |
| **Goals** | | | |
| Plateau pressure | 30 cm $H_2O$ | 30 cm $H_2O$ | – |
| $PaO_2$ | 55–60 mmHg | 55–60 mmHg | 60–80 mmHg |
| pH | 7.2–7.4 | 7.2–7.4 | – |

*For example, at oxygen requirement of 60%, the PEEP should be set at 0.60 x 20, that is 12 cm of $H_2O$.
V-ACMV, volume controlled assist/control mode ventilation; PEEP, positive end-expiratory pressure; $FiO_2$, fraction of inspired oxygen; $PaO_2$, arterial partial pressure of oxygen.

on the spectrum of patients, the financial resources of the organization and the available expertise in handling the equipment. Clearly, the people operating the ventilator are more important than the machine. The choice of a particular mode is often guided by institutional policy or personal preference. In the authors' ICU, ventilation is initiated with volume-controlled ACMV and once the patient improves, the patient is shifted to PSV. As a protocol, we rarely use SIMV for either initial ventilation or later weaning. Newer modes of ventilation are increasingly being promoted to decrease the hazards of conventional ventilation and improve patient-ventilator interactions. However, none of the newer mode of ventilation has been shown superior to conventional modes.[59]

## WEANING FROM MECHANICAL VENTILATION

Weaning is a process of abruptly or gradually withdrawing ventilatory support, and includes discontinuation of mechanical ventilation and removal of artificial airway, if any. The first step in weaning is the assessment of readiness to wean by various clinical, respiratory and hemodynamic parameters (Table 4). Once the patient is deemed ready to be weaned, the commonly used techniques for weaning include SIMV, PSV, and daily spontaneous breathing trials (SBTs). Weaning by SIMV is achieved by gradually decreasing the mandatory breathing rate by 2–4 breaths/minute and allowing the patient for spontaneous breathing effort to maintain the minute ventilation. As traditionally believed, respiratory muscle rest does not occur during mandatory breath of SIMV. In fact, respiratory center

**Table 4: Assessment of Readiness to Wean**

**Clinical parameters**

- Improvement of the underlying cause of respiratory failure
- Awake, alert and cooperative
- No effect of sedation/neuromuscular blockade
- Hemodynamically stable
- Respiratory rate <30 breaths/minute
- Minimal secretions (generally <2 hourly suctioning requirement)

**Ventilatory parameters**

- Spontaneous tidal volume (VT) >5–6 mL/kg
- Vital capacity (VC) >10–12 mL/kg
- PEEP requirement <5 cm of $H_2O$

**Oxygenation criteria**

- $PaCO_2$ <50 mmHg with normal pH
- $PaO_2$ >60 mmHg at $FiO_2$ 0.4 or less
- $SaO_2$ >90% at $FiO_2$ 0.4 or less
- $PaO_2/FiO_2$ >200

output and respiratory muscle activity is as great during the mandatory breaths as the spontaneous breaths.[31,44] The SBT can be performed either with no positive pressure applied to the airway using a T-piece, with a low level of CPAP (5 cm $H_2O$) or a low level of pressure support (PS) (7 cm $H_2O$). Optimal SBT duration has been examined in two studies suggesting that 30 minutes is equivalent to 120 minutes with either T-piece or PSV.[60,61] However, at the authors' institute, an SBT duration of at least 60 minutes is used. Failure of SBT is defined by the presence of tachypnea, tachycardia, arrhythmia, hypertension, hypotension, hypoxemia, or the subjective evidence of agitation or distress, depressed mental status, and diaphoresis.[43,62,63] Gradual reduction of PS is commonly utilized and is the sole mode of mechanical ventilation used during the weaning process in 21% of patients.[64] During weaning, PSV is started at around 10–20 cm of $H_2O$ and reduced by 2–4 cm $H_2O$ at least twice daily till very low values can be tolerated. Recently, gradual reduction of PSV without an initial SBT was found to be associated with better outcomes compared to once daily PSV-supported SBT.[51]

## TROUBLESHOOTING DURING MECHANICAL VENTILATION

Patients experiencing discomfort during mechanical ventilation appear to be in distress, and are anxious, restless, and agitated. There may be dyssynchrony between the patient and the ventilator, i.e., the ventilator appears to be "out of sync" with the patient (also colloquially termed as patient fighting the ventilator), and there may sound several ventilator alarms. An alarm simply signals that there is something wrong with the pressure, volume, flow, or the content of gas being delivered. If the patient appears cyanosed and the physician feels the ventilator is not properly delivering the breaths, the patient should be disconnected from the ventilator, and manually ventilated with 100% oxygen. The common alarms include:

- *High-pressure alarm*: It indicates increased Raw and/or decreased compliance. Common factors associated with increased Raw are the patient biting the endotracheal tube or the airway being blocked by secretions or mucus plug or the underlying obstructive lung disease (asthma, COPD). Patient's cough can also trigger the alarm; however, the ventilator will reset once the cough subsides. A simple way to determine airway patency is to disconnect the ventilator and ventilate the patient with a manual resuscitation bag. High-pressure alarm due to low compliance results from either tension pneumothorax or pulmonary edema (cardiogenic or noncardiogenic). An increase in Ppeak without Pplat suggests increased Raw as the cause of the high-pressure alarm
- *Low-pressure and low-exhaled tidal volume alarms*: It indicates that either the ventilator did not reach the preset pressure or some of the gas that was delivered was not exhaled back into the tubing for measurement. The most common

causes include disconnected tubing or air leaks around the endotracheal tube cuff and poorly secured connections, at the drainage and access ports on the tubing

- *High respiratory rate alarm*: It signals heightened anxiety, awakening from sedation, or pain. This alarm can also occur due to water or kinks in the tubing or from auto-triggering due to inappropriately low trigger-sensitivity
- *Apnea alarm*: It is most commonly due to disconnected tubing, especially where the tubing is attached to the endotracheal tube or tracheostomy tube
- *Low FiO$_2$ alarm*: It arises due to problems with oxygen supply to the ventilator from the mains or due to malfunction of the oxygen-air blender.

## COMPLICATIONS RELATED TO MECHANICAL VENTILATION

The use of mechanical ventilation is associated with several adverse and potentially life-threatening consequences, and the clinician should be aware of these complications as many of these are potentially preventable.

*Complications related to airway intubation*: Intubation may be unduly prolonged, or the right mainstem bronchus may be inadvertently intubated, leading to alveolar hypoventilation or atelectasis, respectively. Cardiac arrhythmias, pulmonary aspiration, and/or significant bleeding may also occur during intubation. Injury to the larynx or trachea can develop while the endotracheal tube is in place.[65,66] Both the tube and its cuff can damage the mucosa, causing edema, inflammation, and/or ulceration. Injury at cuff site is more likely if cuff pressures exceed capillary perfusion pressure (i.e., around 25 cm H$_2$O).[67] Although rare, postintubation tracheal stenosis is the most serious sequel of prolonged intubation.[66,68,69] Mechanical problems such as obstruction of the tube may occur. Cuff leaks may also develop, increasing the risk of pulmonary aspiration. Accidental extubation may occur in about 10% of patients.[70]

The most important complication of an artificial airway is the development of lower respiratory tract infection, the so-called VAP.[71] It is defined as the appearance of a new radiographic infiltrate appearing at least 48 hours after induction of mechanical ventilation. The oropharynx and the gastrointestinal tract of mechanically ventilated patients are colonized by pathogenic bacteria, and the endotracheal tube allows potential pathogens to enter the trachea. Other contributing factors include ventilator circuit, respiratory therapy equipment, hands of medical personnel, disruption of coughing mechanism and mucociliary escalator. Various methods have been proposed to reduce the risk of VAP (Table 5).

*Complications related to invasive ventilation*: Positive pressure ventilation may lead to several complications, the most important of which are VALI, barotrauma, oxygen toxicity, and adverse cardiovascular consequences. VALI is lung injury that

<table>
<tr><td>Table 5: Preventive Strategies for Ventilator-associated Pneumonia</td></tr>
</table>

- Head end elevation to 30–45°
- Oral cavity decontamination with 2% chlorhexidine[72-75]
- Hand hygiene preferably using alcohol-based hand rubs or soap and water[76]
- Use of sedation and weaning protocols[77,78]
- Use of noninvasive to avoid intubation, where feasible[79,80]
- Subglottic secretion drainage[81,82]
- Heat and moisture exchangers in place of heated humidifiers[83-87]
- Closed suction systems[88-90]
- Use of orotracheal intubation as opposed to nasotracheal intubation[91,92]
- Proper and timely disposal of condensates[93,94]
- Maintaining tracheal cuff pressures <25 cm $H_2O$[95]
- Wipe stethoscopes with alcohol rubs[96]
- Proper sterilization of nebulizer and other chambers

develops as a consequence of mechanical ventilation. The proposed mechanisms include overdistension of the alveoli due to high VTs (volutrauma), cyclical opening and closing of the alveoli (atelectotrauma), and release of inflammatory mediators due to overdistension (biotrauma).[97] The recognition of VALI has resulted in lung-protective ventilatory strategies including limiting the VT to 6 mL/kg, even in the normal lung. Pulmonary barotrauma is the presence of extra-alveolar air, and includes pneumothorax, pneumomediastinum, pneumopericardium, pneumoperitoneum, and interstitial and subcutaneous emphysema. Incidence of barotrauma is variable, with most studies reporting figures of 5–15%.[98] The presence of severe underlying lung disease, necrotizing pneumonia, ARDS, and high airway pressures markedly increase the risk for this complication.[99] Strategies that prevent the exposure of lung to high pressures (limiting overdistension) may be associated with less barotrauma. Such approaches include PCV and pressure-limited, volume-cycled ventilation. Human pulmonary oxygen toxicity varies from subclinical cellular changes to clinical manifestations of tracheobronchitis, absorption atelectasis, noncardiogenic pulmonary edema, and pulmonary fibrosis. Both capillary endothelial and alveolar epithelial cells are damaged due to oxidant injury related to excessive free radical generation. Besides, several extrapulmonary adverse effects can also occur due to hyperoxia such as increased systemic vascular resistance, bradycardia, headache, nausea, vomiting, and hypesthesia. Oxygen toxicity can be easily prevented by maintaining $FiO_2$ at less than 0.5–0.6.[100]

The hemodynamic consequences of mechanical ventilation result from positive airway pressure transmitted to the pleural space, heart and great vessels within the chest. Positive Ppl decreases venous return, right ventricular preload, and left ventricular afterload.[101,102] Left ventricular compliance may be reduced due to the compressive effect of hyperinflated lungs.[103] All these factors, along with endocardial ischemia, contribute to a diminished cardiac output and hypotension.

*Other complications*: Positive pressure ventilation causes a reduction in urine output and retention of salt and water. Sympathetic activation due to a reduction in cardiac output constricts afferent renal arterioles and causes a redistribution of blood flow from cortical to juxtamedullary nephrons, thereby reducing glomerular filtration rate and urinary sodium excretion. Activation of the renin-angiotensin-aldosterone system (due to decreased renal blood flow) as well as inhibition of atrial natriuretic peptide release (due to reduction in left atrial stretch) further aggravates these changes. Plasma arginine vasopressin (AVP) is also increased, due either to a baroreceptor discharge following a decrease of transmural aortic pressure or to the response of atrial stretch receptors to a decrease in thoracic blood volume. AVP acts both as a vasoconstrictor and an antidiuretic agent and decreases free water clearance. Finally, an increase in inferior vena caval and renal vein pressures may decrease renal blood flow as well. The net effect of all these factors is salt and water retention with decreased urine output.

Critically ill patients are predisposed to increased risk of gastrointestinal hemorrhage, primarily from stress ulcers. The incidence varies from 6 to 30% in several studies,[104] and may be even higher in patients with ARDS or multiorgan failure. Pathogenesis of stress ulcer formation is multifactorial and related to low intraluminal gastric pH, gastric mucosal ischemia secondary to splanchnic hypoperfusion, impaired ability to repair damaged tissue, and bile salt regurgitation. Stress ulcer prophylaxis is nowadays routinely given to all ventilated patients.[105]

Increased intrathoracic pressure can elevate jugular venous and intracranial pressures, and thereby reduce cerebral perfusion pressures. Tracheal suctioning may also be associated with a rise in intracranial pressure. Such effects assume particular importance in the setting of reduce mean arterial pressures and reduced intracranial compliance resulting from head injury or neurosurgical intervention.[106] Patients with normal intracranial pressure do not appear to develop such complications.

*Adverse effects of sedation and paralysis*: Neuromuscular paralysis and/or sedation are often required to allow patient comfort and facilitate invasive ventilation. Sedation may result in vasodilatation that contributes to hypotension and diminished cardiac output. Paralytic agents immobilize patients, encouraging retention of secretions, atelectasis and muscle wasting. Neuromuscular blocking agents are associated with an acute myopathy that causes muscle weakness to persist long after withdrawal of drug treatment.[107] The risk of critical illness neuromuscular abnormality is as high as 50% in ICU patients with protracted mechanical ventilation.

*Equipment malfunction*: There is paucity of information on morbidity and mortality resulting from failure of ventilator and/or respiratory therapy equipment. The problems attributable to ventilator malfunction include mechanical failure of ventilator, alarm failure, overheating of inspired air, alarms left inadvertently in "off" position, and inadequate nebulization or humidification.[108,109] In one study, 37% of all complications were related to equipment malfunction, and 48% of these resulted in significant morbidity.[110] While the ventilator is a dependable equipment, good alarm systems and sophisticated surveillance systems are beneficial, they cannot replace careful monitoring by trained personnel.

## CONCLUSION

The purpose of mechanical ventilation is to provide assisted ventilation to a patient with respiratory failure. Recent advances in the knowledge of VALI have forced major revisions in our approach to ventilatory support. Thus, correction of gas exchange is no longer the only objective; equal emphasis is now being placed on prevention of lung injury and other ventilator-associated complications. Newer modes of mechanical ventilation and ventilators present alternate options for supporting patients with respiratory failure, but their clinical efficacy still remains to be proven.

### Editor's Comment

*Mechanical ventilation is an integral part of any intensive care unit (ICU). From an era of crude ventilatory support, we have come into a time where highly sophisticated computerized ventilators have entered the market. Along with better ventilation, our understanding of the benefits and harms associated with ventilation has also increased tremendously. A number of very well conducted studies by the Acute Respiratory Distress Syndrome Network have changed the way ventilator support is being given today. Initially, a concept of high tidal volume was almost universal in the ICU. We have now come to accept that this can be harmful and is associated with high mortality, and low tidal volume strategy for ventilation is now well established. Also, the complications that occur with current assisted ventilation have become more defined. This has led to a well-established evidence-based guidelines for the use of noninvasive ventilation in some situations. Although a lot of sophistication has occurred in the technology of ventilators, the basic modes of ventilation are still the same and for many beginners it is important to understand these well. It is debatable how significant the newer modes of ventilation have improved morbidity and mortality. The challenge that still remains is to prevent ventilator associated complications especially infections.*

***Randeep Guleria***

# REFERENCES


1. Slutsky AS. History of mechanical ventilation. From Vesalius to ventilator-induced lung injury. *Am J Respir Crit Care Med.* 2015;191(10):1106-15.
2. Ibsen B. The anaesthetist's viewpoint on the treatment of respiratory complications in poliomyelitis during the epidemic in Copenhagen, 1952. *Proc R Soc Med.* 1954;47(1):72-4.
3. Garland A, Gershengorn HB. Staffing in ICUs: physicians and alternative staffing models. *Chest.* 2013;143(1):214-21.
4. Agarwal R, Aggarwal AN, Gupta D. Is noninvasive pressure support ventilation as effective and safe as continuous positive airway pressure in cardiogenic pulmonary oedema? *Singapore Med J.* 2009;50(6):595-603.
5. Agarwal R, Aggarwal AN, Gupta D. Role of noninvasive ventilation in acute lung injury/acute respiratory distress syndrome: a proportion meta-analysis. *Respir Care.* 2010;55(12):1653-60.
6. Agarwal R, Aggarwal AN, Gupta D, Jindal SK. Non-invasive ventilation in acute cardiogenic pulmonary oedema. *Postgrad Med J.* 2005;81(960):637-43.
7. Agarwal R, Gupta D. What is the role of noninvasive ventilation in diastolic heart failure? *Intensive Care Med.* 2005;31(10):1451; author reply 1452.
8. Agarwal R, Gupta D, Handa A, Aggarwal AN. Noninvasive ventilation in ARDS caused by *Mycobacterium tuberculosis*: report of three cases and review of literature. *Intensive Care Med.* 2005;31(12):1723-4.
9. Agarwal R, Handa A, Aggarwal AN, Gupta D, Behera D. Outcomes of noninvasive ventilation in acute hypoxemic respiratory failure in a respiratory intensive care unit in north India. *Respir Care.* 2009;54(12):1679-87.
10. Slutsky AS. Mechanical ventilation. American College of Chest Physicians' Consensus Conference. *Chest.* 1993;104(6):1833-59.
11. Ceriana P, Nava S. Hypoxic and hypercapnic respiratory failure. *Eur Respir Mon.* 2006;36:1-15.
12. Gnanapandithan K, Agarwal R. Respiratory Failure. In: Jindal SK, Shankar PS, Gupta D, Raoof S, Aggarwal AN, Agarwal R (Eds). Textbook of Pulmonary and Critical Care Medicine, 1st edition. New Delhi: Jaypee Brothers Medical Publishers (P) Ltd.; 2011. pp. 1609-17.
13. Ventilation with lower tidal volumes as compared with traditional tidal volumes for acute lung injury and the acute respiratory distress syndrome. The Acute Respiratory Distress Syndrome Network. *N Engl J Med.* 2000;342(18):1301-8.
14. Gama de Abreu M, Heintz M, Heller A, Széchényi R, Albrecht DM, Koch T. One-lung ventilation with high tidal volumes and zero positive end-expiratory pressure is injurious in the isolated rabbit lung model. *Anesth Analg.* 2003;96(1):220-8, table of contents.
15. Choi G, Wolthuis EK, Bresser P, Levi M, van der Poll T, Dzoljic M, et al. Mechanical ventilation with lower tidal volumes and positive end-expiratory pressure prevents alveolar coagulation in patients without lung injury. *Anesthesiology.* 2006;105(4):689-95.
16. Mascia L, Zavala E, Bosma K, Pasero D, Decaroli D, Andrews P, et al. High tidal volume is associated with the development of acute lung injury after severe brain injury: an international observational study. *Crit Care Med.* 2007;35(8):1815-20.
17. Yilmaz M, Keegan MT, Iscimen R, Afessa B, Buck CF, Hubmayr RD, et al. Toward the prevention of acute lung injury: protocol-guided limitation of large tidal volume ventilation and inappropriate transfusion. *Crit Care Med.* 2007;35(7):1660-6; quiz 1667.
18. Meier T, Lange A, Papenberg H, Ziemann M, Fentrop C, Uhlig U, et al. Pulmonary cytokine responses during mechanical ventilation of noninjured lungs with and without end-expiratory pressure. *Anesth Analg.* 2008;107(4):1265-75.
19. Wolthuis EK, Choi G, Dessing MC, Bresser P, Lutter R, Dzoljic M, et al. Mechanical ventilation with lower tidal volumes and positive end-expiratory pressure prevents pulmonary inflammation in patients without preexisting lung injury. *Anesthesiology.* 2008;108(1):46-54.
20. Determann RM, Royakkers A, Wolthuis EK, Vlaar AP, Choi G, Paulus F, et al. Ventilation with lower tidal volumes as compared with conventional tidal volumes for patients without acute lung injury: a preventive randomized controlled trial. *Crit Care.* 2010;14(1):R1.

21. Hong CM, Xu DZ, Lu Q, Cheng Y, Pisarenko V, Doucet D, et al. Low tidal volume and high positive end-expiratory pressure mechanical ventilation results in increased inflammation and ventilator-associated lung injury in normal lungs. *Anesth Analg.* 2010;110(6):1652-60.

22. Weingarten TN, Whalen FX, Warner DO, Gajic O, Schears GJ, Snyder MR, et al. Comparison of two ventilatory strategies in elderly patients undergoing major abdominal surgery. *Br J Anaesth.* 2010;104(1):16-22.

23. Serpa Neto A, Cardoso SO, Manetta JA, Pereira VG, Espósito DC, Pasqualucci Mde O, et al. Association between use of lung-protective ventilation with lower tidal volumes and clinical outcomes among patients without acute respiratory distress syndrome: a meta-analysis. *JAMA.* 2012;308(16):1651-9.

24. Gu WJ, Wang F, Liu JC. Effect of lung-protective ventilation with lower tidal volumes on clinical outcomes among patients undergoing surgery: a meta-analysis of randomized controlled trials. *CMAJ.* 2015;187(3):E101-9.

25. Gupta D, Jindal SK. Complications of oxygen therapy. In: Jindal SK, Agarwal R (Eds). Oxygen Therapy, 2nd edition. New Delhi: Jaypee Brothers Medical Publishers (P) Ltd.; 2008. pp. 254-68.

26. Vargas M, Sutherasan Y, Gregoretti C, Pelosi P. PEEP role in ICU and operating room: from pathophysiology to clinical practice. *ScientificWorldJournal.* 2014;2014:852356.

27. Marini JJ. Dynamic hyperinflation and auto-positive end-expiratory pressure: lessons learned over 30 years. *Am J Respir Crit Care Med.* 2011;184(7):756-62.

28. Ranieri VM, Grasso S, Fiore T, Giuliani R. Auto-positive end-expiratory pressure and dynamic hyperinflation. *Clin Chest Med.* 1996;17(3):379-94.

29. Pepe PE, Marini JJ. Occult positive end-expiratory pressure in mechanically ventilated patients with airflow obstruction: the auto-PEEP effect. *Am Rev Respir Dis.* 1982;126(1):166-70.

30. Connors AF Jr, McCaffree DR, Gray BA. Effect of inspiratory flow rate on gas exchange during mechanical ventilation. *Am Rev Respir Dis.* 1981;124(5):537-43.

31. Imsand C, Feihl F, Perret C, Fitting JW. Regulation of inspiratory neuromuscular output during synchronized intermittent mechanical ventilation. *Anesthesiology.* 1994;80(1):13-22.

32. Marini JJ, Ravenscraft SA. Mean airway pressure: physiologic determinants and clinical importance—Part 1: Physiologic determinants and measurements. *Crit Care Med.* 1992;20(10):1461-72.

33. Marini JJ, Ravenscraft SA. Mean airway pressure: physiologic determinants and clinical importance—Part 2: Clinical implications. *Crit Care Med.* 1992;20(11):1604-16.

34. Jonson B, Svantesson C. Elastic pressure-volume curves: what information do they convey? *Thorax.* 1999;54(1):82-7.

35. Gattinoni L, Pelosi P, Suter PM, Pedoto A, Vercesi P, Lissoni A. Acute respiratory distress syndrome caused by pulmonary and extrapulmonary disease. Different syndromes? *Am J Respir Crit Care Med.* 1998;158(1):3-11.

36. Talmor D, Sarge T, O'Donnell CR, Ritz R, Malhotra A, Lisbon A, et al. Esophageal and transpulmonary pressures in acute respiratory failure. *Crit Care Med.* 2006;34(5):1389-94.

37. D'Angelo E, Robatto FM, Calderini E, Tavola M, Bono D, Torri G, et al. Pulmonary and chest wall mechanics in anesthetized paralyzed humans. *J Appl Physiol.* 1991;70(6):2602-10.

38. McIlroy MB, Tierney DF, Nadel JA. A new method for measurement of compliance and resistance of lungs and thorax. *J Appl Physiol.* 1963;18(2):424-7.

39. Chatburn RL. A new system for understanding mechanical ventilators. *Respir Care.* 1991;36(10):1123-55.

40. Chatburn RL, Primiano FP Jr. A new system for understanding modes of mechanical ventilation. *Respir Care.* 2001;46(6):604-21.

41. Chatburn RL. Classification of ventilator modes: update and proposal for implementation. *Respir Care.* 2007;52(3):301-23.

42. Chatburn RL, El-Khatib M, Mireles-Cabodevila E. A taxonomy for mechanical ventilation: 10 fundamental maxims. *Respir Care.* 2014;59(11):1747-63.

43. Esteban A, Frutos F, Tobin MJ, Alía I, Solsona JF, Vallverdú I, et al. A comparison of four methods of weaning patients from mechanical ventilation. Spanish Lung Failure Collaborative Group. *N Engl J Med.* 1995;332(6):345-50.

44. Marini JJ, Smith TC, Lamb VJ. External work output and force generation during synchronized intermittent mechanical ventilation. Effect of machine assistance on breathing effort. *Am Rev Respir Dis.* 1988;138(5):1169-79.

45. Sassoon CS, Del Rosario N, Fei R, Rheeman CH, Gruer SE, Mahutte CK. Influence of pressure- and flow-triggered synchronous intermittent mandatory ventilation on inspiratory muscle work. *Crit Care Med.* 1994;22(12):1933-41.

46. Leung P, Jubran A, Tobin MJ. Comparison of assisted ventilator modes on triggering, patient effort, and dyspnea. *Am J Respir Crit Care Med.* 1997;155(6):1940-8.

47. Hess DR. Ventilator modes: where have we come from and where are we going? *Chest.* 2010;137(6):1256-8.

48. MacIntyre NR. Respiratory function during pressure support ventilation. *Chest.* 1986;89(5):677-83.

49. Fiastro JF, Habib MP, Quan SF. Pressure support compensation for inspiratory work due to endotracheal tubes and demand continuous positive airway pressure. *Chest.* 1988;93(3):499-505.

50. Aggarwal AN, Agarwal R, Gupta D. Automatic tube compensation as an adjunct for weaning in patients with severe neuroparalytic snake envenomation requiring mechanical ventilation: a pilot randomized study. *Respir Care.* 2009;54(12):1697-702.

51. Gnanapandithan K, Agarwal R, Aggarwal AN, Gupta D. Weaning by gradual pressure support (PS) reduction without an initial spontaneous breathing trial (SBT) versus PS-supported SBT: a pilot study. *Rev Port Pneumol.* 2011;17(6):244-52.

52. Chatburn RL, Mireles-Cabodevila E. Closed-loop control of mechanical ventilation: description and classification of targeting schemes. *Respir Care.* 2011;56(1):85-102.

53. Agarwal R, Gupta R, Aggarwal AN, Gupta D. Noninvasive positive pressure ventilation in acute respiratory failure due to COPD vs. other causes: effectiveness and predictors of failure in a respiratory ICU in North India. *Int J Chron Obstruct Pulmon Dis.* 2008;3(4):737-43.

54. Agarwal R. Noninvasive ventilation in acute lung injury/acute respiratory distress syndrome. In: Esquinas AM (Ed). Noninvasive Mechanical Ventilation: Theory, Equipment, and Clinical Applications. Berlin: Springer; 2010. pp. 241-8.

55. Agarwal R, Reddy C, Aggarwal AN, Gupta D. Is there a role for noninvasive ventilation in acute respiratory distress syndrome? A meta-analysis. *Respir Med.* 2006;100(12):2235-8.

56. Gupta D, Nath A, Agarwal R, Behera D. A prospective randomized controlled trial on the efficacy of noninvasive ventilation in severe acute asthma. *Respir Care.* 2010;55(5):536-43.

57. Mead J, Takishima T, Leith D. Stress distribution in lungs: a model of pulmonary elasticity. *J Appl Physiol.* 1970;28(5):596-608.

58. Hickling KG, Henderson SJ, Jackson R. Low mortality associated with low volume pressure limited ventilation with permissive hypercapnia in severe adult respiratory distress syndrome. *Intensive Care Med.* 1990;16(6):372-7.

59. Agarwal R, Srinivasan A, Aggarwal AN, Gupta D. Adaptive support ventilation for complete ventilatory support in acute respiratory distress syndrome: a pilot, randomized controlled trial. *Respirology.* 2013;18(7):1108-15.

60. Esteban A, Alia I, Tobin MJ, Gil A, Gordo F, Vallverdú I, et al. Effect of spontaneous breathing trial duration on outcome of attempts to discontinue mechanical ventilation. Spanish Lung Failure Collaborative Group. *Am J Respir Crit Care Med.* 1999;159(2):512-8.

61. Perren A, Domenighetti G, Mauri S, Genini F, Vizzardi N. Protocol-directed weaning from mechanical ventilation: clinical outcome in patients randomized for a 30-min or 120-min trial with pressure support ventilation. *Intensive Care Med.* 2002;28(8):1058-63.

62. Brochard L, Rauss A, Benito S, Conti G, Mancebo J, Rekik N, et al. Comparison of three methods of gradual withdrawal from ventilatory support during weaning from mechanical ventilation. *Am J Respir Crit Care Med.* 1994;150(4):896-903.

63. Vallverdú I, Calaf N, Subirana M, Net A, Benito S, Mancebo J. Clinical characteristics, respiratory functional parameters, and outcome of a two-hour T-piece trial in patients weaning from mechanical ventilation. *Am J Respir Crit Care Med.* 1998;158(6):1855-62.

64. Esteban A, Anzueto A, Frutos F, Alía I, Brochard L, Stewart TE, et al. Characteristics and outcomes in adult patients receiving mechanical ventilation: a 28-day international study. *JAMA.* 2002;287(3):345-55.

65. Stone DJ, Bogdonoff DL. Airway considerations in the management of patients requiring long-term endotracheal intubation. *Anesth Analg.* 1992;74(2):276-87.

66. Colice GL, Stukel TA, Dain B. Laryngeal complications of prolonged intubation. *Chest.* 1989;96(4):877-84.

67. Bishop MJ. Mechanisms of laryngotracheal injury following prolonged tracheal intubation. *Chest.* 1989;96(1):185-6.

68. Agarwal R, Khan A, Aggarwal AN, Singh N, Bhagat H, Kumar B, et al. Initial experience of endobronchial silicon stents from a tertiary care centre in North India. *Indian J Chest Dis Allied Sci.* 2011;53(2):93-8.

69. Madan K, Agarwal R, Aggarwal AN, Gupta D. Therapeutic rigid bronchoscopy at a tertiary care center in North India: initial experience and systematic review of Indian literature. *Lung India.* 2014;31(1):9-15.

70. Boulain T. Unplanned extubations in the adult intensive care unit: a prospective multicenter study. Association des Reanimateurs du Centre-Ouest. *Am J Respir Crit Care Med.* 1998;157(4 Pt 1):1131-7.

71. Gupta D, Agarwal R, Aggarwal AN, Singh N, Mishra N, Khilnani GC, et al. Guidelines for diagnosis and management of community- and hospital-acquired pneumonia in adults: Joint ICS/NCCP(I) recommendations. *Lung India.* 2012;29(Suppl 2):S27-62.

72. Tantipong H, Morkchareonpong C, Jaiyindee S, Thamlikitkul V. Randomized controlled trial and meta-analysis of oral decontamination with 2% chlorhexidine solution for the prevention of ventilator-associated pneumonia. *Infect Control Hosp Epidemiol.* 2008;29(2):131-6.

73. Zamora Zamora F. Effectiveness of oral care in the prevention of ventilator-associated pneumonia. systematic review and meta-analysis of randomised clinical trials. *Enferm Clin.* 2011;21(6):308-19.

74. Chan EY, Ruest A, Meade MO, Cook DJ. Oral decontamination for prevention of pneumonia in mechanically ventilated adults: systematic review and meta-analysis. *BMJ.* 2007;334(7599):889.

75. Chlebicki MP, Safdar N. Topical chlorhexidine for prevention of ventilator-associated pneumonia: a meta-analysis. *Crit Care Med.* 2007;35(2):595-602.

76. Rabie T, Curtis V. Handwashing and risk of respiratory infections: a quantitative systematic review. *Trop Med Int Health.* 2006;11(3):258-67.

77. Girard TD, Kress JP, Fuchs BD, Thomason JW, Schweickert WD, Pun BT, et al. Efficacy and safety of a paired sedation and ventilator weaning protocol for mechanically ventilated patients in intensive care (Awakening and Breathing Controlled trial): a randomised controlled trial. *Lancet.* 2008;371(9607):126-34.

78. Robertson TE, Mann HJ, Hyzy R, Rogers A, Douglas I, Waxman AB, et al. Multicenter implementation of a consensus-developed, evidence-based, spontaneous breathing trial protocol. *Crit Care Med.* 2008;36(10):2753-62.

79. Nourdine K, Combes P, Carton MJ, Beuret P, Cannamela A, Ducreux JC. Does noninvasive ventilation reduce the ICU nosocomial infection risk? A prospective clinical survey. *Intensive Care Med.* 1999;25(6):567-73.

80. Girou E, Schortgen F, Delclaux C, Brun-Buisson C, Blot F, Lefort Y, et al. Association of noninvasive ventilation with nosocomial infections and survival in critically ill patients. *JAMA.* 2000;284(18):2361-7.

81. Bouza E, Perez MJ, Munoz P, Rincon C, Barrio JM, Hortal J. Continuous aspiration of subglottic secretions in the prevention of ventilator-associated pneumonia in the postoperative period of major heart surgery. *Chest.* 2008;134(5):938-46.

82. Dezfulian C, Shojania K, Collard HR, Kim HM, Matthay MA, Saint S. Subglottic secretion drainage for preventing ventilator-associated pneumonia: a meta-analysis. *Am J Med.* 2005;118(1):11-8.

83. Boots RJ, George N, Faoagali JL, Druery J, Dean K, Heller RF. Double-heater-wire circuits and heat-and-moisture exchangers and the risk of ventilator-associated pneumonia. *Crit Care Med.* 2006;34(3):687-93.

84. Bench S. Humidification in the long-term ventilated patient: a systematic review. *Intensive Crit Care Nurs.* 2003;19(2):75-84.

85. Lorente L, Lecuona M, Jimenez A, Mora ML, Sierra A. Ventilator-associated pneumonia using a heated humidifier or a heat and moisture exchanger: a randomized controlled trial (ISRCTN88724583). *Crit Care.* 2006;10(4):R116.

86. Ricard JD, Boyer A, Dreyfuss D. The effect of humidification on the incidence of ventilator-associated pneumonia. *Respir Care Clin N Am.* 2006;12(2):263-73.

87. Lacherade JC, Auburtin M, Cerf C, Van de Louw A, Soufir L, Rebufat Y, et al. Impact of humidification systems on ventilator-associated pneumonia: a randomized multicenter trial. *Am J Respir Crit Care Med.* 2005;172(10):1276-82.

88. Subirana M, Sola I, Benito S. Closed tracheal suction systems versus open tracheal suction systems for mechanically ventilated adult patients. *Cochrane Database Syst Rev.* 2007;(4):CD004581.

89. Harada N. Closed suctioning system: critical analysis for its use. *Jpn J Nurs Sci.* 2010;7(1):19-28.

90. Siempos II, Vardakas KZ, Falagas ME. Closed tracheal suction systems for prevention of ventilator-associated pneumonia. *Br J Anaesth.* 2008;100(3):299-306.

91. Holzapfel L, Chastang C, Demingeon G, Bohe J, Piralla B, Coupry A. A randomized study assessing the systematic search for maxillary sinusitis in nasotracheally mechanically ventilated patients. Influence of nosocomial maxillary sinusitis on the occurrence of ventilator-associated pneumonia. *Am J Respir Crit Care Med.* 1999;159(3):695-701.

92. Holzapfel L, Chevret S, Madinier G, Ohen F, Demingeon G, Coupry A, et al. Influence of long-term oro- or nasotracheal intubation on nosocomial maxillary sinusitis and pneumonia: results of a prospective, randomized, clinical trial. *Crit Care Med.* 1993;21(8):1132-8.

93. Craven DE, Goularte TA, Make BJ. Contaminated condensate in mechanical ventilator circuits. A risk factor for nosocomial pneumonia? *Am Rev Respir Dis.* 1984;129(4):625-8.

94. Craven DE, Lichtenberg DA, Goularte TA, Make BJ, McCabe WR. Contaminated medication nebulizers in mechanical ventilator circuits. Source of bacterial aerosols. *Am J Med.* 1984;77(5):834-8.

95. Rello J, Soñora R, Jubert P, Artigas A, Rué M, Vallés J. Pneumonia in intubated patients: role of respiratory airway care. *Am J Respir Crit Care Med.* 1996;154(1):111-5.

96. Mehta AK, Halvosa JS, Gould CV, Steinberg JP. Efficacy of alcohol-based hand rubs in the disinfection of stethoscopes. *Infect Control Hosp Epidemiol.* 2010;31(8):870-2.

97. Slutsky AS, Ranieri VM. Ventilator-induced lung injury. *N Engl J Med.* 2013;369(22):2126-36.

98. Gammon RB, Shin MS, Buchalter SE. Pulmonary barotrauma in mechanical ventilation. Patterns and risk factors. *Chest.* 1992;102(2):568-72.

99. Haake R, Schlichtig R, Ulstad DR, Henschen RR. Barotrauma. Pathophysiology, risk factors, and prevention. *Chest.* 1987;91(4):608-13.

100. Deneke SM, Fanburg BL. Normobaric oxygen toxicity of the lung. *N Engl J Med.* 1980;303(2):76-86.

101. Robotham JL, Lixfeld W, Holland L, MacGregor D, Bromberger-Barnea B, Permutt S, et al. The effects of positive end-expiratory pressure on right and left ventricular performance. *Am Rev Respir Dis.* 1980;121(4):677-83.

102. Abel JG, Salerno TA, Panos A, Greyson ND, Rice TW, Teoh K, et al. Cardiovascular effects of positive pressure ventilation in humans. *Ann Thorac Surg.* 1987;43(2):198-206.

103. Leithner C, Podolsky A, Globits S, Frank H, Neuhold A, Pidlich J, et al. Magnetic resonance imaging of the heart during positive end-expiratory pressure ventilation in normal subjects. *Crit Care Med.* 1994;22(3):426-32.

104. Marik PE, Vasu T, Hirani A, Pachinburavan M. Stress ulcer prophylaxis in the new millennium: a systematic review and meta-analysis. *Crit Care Med.* 2010;38(11):2222-8.

105. Alhazzani W, Alenezi F, Jaeschke RZ, Moayyedi P, Cook DJ. Proton pump inhibitors versus histamine 2 receptor antagonists for stress ulcer prophylaxis in critically ill patients: a systematic review and meta-analysis. *Crit Care Med.* 2013;41(3):693-705.

106. Gemma M, Tommasino C, Cerri M, Giannotti A, Piazzi B, Borghi T. Intracranial effects of endotracheal suctioning in the acute phase of head injury. *J Neurosurg Anesthesiol.* 2002;14(1):50-4.

107. Stevens RD, Dowdy DW, Michaels RK, Mendez-Tellez PA, Pronovost PJ, Needham DM. Neuromuscular dysfunction acquired in critical illness: a systematic review. *Intensive Care Med.* 2007;33(11):1876-91.

108. Feeley TW, Bancroft ML. Problems with mechanical ventilators. *Int Anesthesiol Clin.* 1982;20(3):83-93.

109. Zwillich CW, Pierson DJ, Creagh CE, Sutton FD, Schatz E, Petty TL. Complications of assisted ventilation. A prospective study of 354 consecutive episodes. *Am J Med.* 1974;57(2):161-70.

110. Abramson NS, Wald KS, Grenvik AN, Robinson D, Snyder JV. Adverse occurrences in intensive care units. *JAMA.* 1980;244(14):1582-4.

World Clin Pulm Crit Care Med. 2016;4(1):36-47.

# Weaning from Assisted Ventilation

Saurabh Mittal MD, *Karan Madan MD DM

Department of Pulmonary Medicine and Sleep Disorders, All India Institute of Medical Sciences
New Delhi, India

## ABSTRACT

Weaning from assisted ventilation is a gradual process of resumption of spontaneous breathing. More than half the time spent in intensive care unit is spent in weaning process. Weaning process should start as soon as patient is initiated on assisted ventilation. Readiness to wean should be assessed daily in all patients by looking at primary disease status, hemodynamic status, metabolic parameters, and sensorium. Multiple studies have shown that sedation-free interval and daily spontaneous awakening trial helps in early weaning. Various methods for spontaneous breathing trial (SBT) include pressure support ventilation, continuous positive airway pressure, and T-piece trial. None of these methods have been found to be superior to each other and all have almost equal predictability for successful weaning. A 30-minute SBT has been found noninferior to 120-minute SBT. The two other important parameters to assess before extubation include: (i) cuff leak test to predict postextubation laryngeal edema and (ii) assessment for patient's ability to handle secretions. Elderly age, multiple comorbidities, and morbid obesity are few of the factors that predict extubation failure. Many indices like maximum inspiratory pressure (PImax), P0.1, P0.1/PImax and CROP (compliance, rate, oxygenation, pressure) index have been studied and may be useful to predict successful weaning. Newer modes of ventilation like proportional assist ventilation, adaptive servo-ventilation, and neurally adjusted ventilatory assist may be useful when a patient with difficult weaning is encountered. Early and comprehensive assessment for weaning remains the key to successful weaning and postextubation monitoring is essential to improve patient outcome.

*Corresponding author
*Email:* drkaranmadan@gmail.com

## INTRODUCTION

Mechanical ventilation is an important event in the care of patients with respiratory failure due to various etiologies. Though life saving, its inherent multitude complications make its discontinuation at the earliest desirable. Weaning is an important part of critical care and requires continuous effort from the intensivist and patient cooperation for a successful outcome. It requires an aggressive approach from critical care team for earliest possible discontinuation of mechanical ventilation.

Weaning constitutes the gradual withdrawal of mechanical ventilation and the resumption of spontaneous breathing. It includes two processes, i.e., discontinuation of mechanical ventilation and removal of endotracheal tube. Since the ultimate goal is to liberate the patient from mechanical ventilation and not in all patients does the process need to be gradual, the term "liberation from mechanical ventilation" is preferred over "weaning".[1] Around 40–50% of total duration of mechanical ventilation is spent during the process of weaning. A delay in weaning is associated with the risk of increased mortality and other complications of mechanical ventilation like ventilator-associated pneumonia (VAP). To minimize the morbidity, mortality, and healthcare costs, early successful weaning should be the target of critical care. Meanwhile, it is of utmost importance to avoid weaning failures and reintubations which carry their own risks.[2]

## WEANING PROCESS

The weaning process should begin as soon as possible. It begins with the recognition by the clinician of the probability of a successful weaning. This is generally after the underlying cause for respiratory failure is treated or improving. Once this stage is reached, the readiness of the patient for weaning is assessed by well established subjective and objective criteria referred to as the "wean screen"[2] (Table 1).

Discontinuation of sedation and daily spontaneous awakening trial is an important step in the weaning process. Continuous intravenous sedation has been found to be associated with increased duration of mechanical ventilation.[3] Many trials have shown the utility of daily interruption of sedation and awakening trial in reducing the duration of ventilation, facilitating weaning and reducing the length of intensive care unit (ICU) stay.[4]

### How to Assess Rapid Shallow Breathing Index

It was observed that patients who fail a spontaneous breathing trial (SBT) are more likely to develop rapid and shallow breathing than those who succeed. Rapid shallow breathing index (RSBI) has been extensively studied as a predictor of weaning and is found to be better than other predictors of weaning outcome. After 1 minute of unassisted breathing, measure respiratory rate (RR) and minute

| **Table 1: Parameters to Assess Readiness to Wean** | |
| --- | --- |
| Subjective assessment | • Adequate cough reflex |
| | • Absence of excessive tracheobronchial secretions |
| | • Resolution of or improving disease state for which the patient was intubated |
| Clinical stability | • Stable cardiovascular and metabolic status (including serum electrolytes especially $K^+$, $Mg^{++}$, and $PO_4^{---}$) |
| | • HR <140 bpm |
| | • Systolic BP 90–160 mmHg on no or minimal vasopressors |
| Adequate oxygenation | • $SaO_2$ >90% on $FiO_2$ <0.4 |
| | • PEEP <8 cm $H_2O$ |
| Adequate pulmonary function | • Respiratory rate <35 bpm |
| | • Tidal volume >5 mL/kg |
| | • Respiratory rate/tidal volume (RSBI) <105 breaths/min/L |
| | • No significant respiratory acidosis |
| Adequate mentation | • No sedation |

HR, heart rate; BP, blood pressure, PEEP, positive end-expiratory pressure; RSBI, rapid shallow breathing index.

ventilation for 1 minute during unassisted breathing: [0 positive end-expiratory pressure (PEEP)/5 cm $H_2O$ pressure support ventilation (PSV)]. At the end of 1 minute divide the minute ventilation by RR to calculate the average tidal volume (VT). Then divide the RR by the VT to obtain the RSBI.

## SPONTANEOUS BREATHING TRIAL

Once the patient satisfies the above criteria, ability to breathe spontaneously is assessed by SBT. There have been various methods used to give SBT to patients which include PSV, continuous PEEP, or ventilation via a T-piece. No significant difference was observed between SBT using a T-tube and pressure support of 7 cm $H_2O$.[5] Initially SBT was given for 2 hours but it has been shown that a 30-minute trial is equivalent to a 2-hour SBT in predicting weaning success.[6]

Spontaneous breathing trial failure is identified by the following parameters though they are not absolute and individual discretion should be used by clinicians while assessing the same (Table 2).

Nearly 70% of the patients tolerate the first SBT and are extubated successfully termed "simple weaning". They have a good prognosis with a low ICU and in-hospital mortality. Other groups of patients have a "difficult weaning" requiring up to 3 SBTs but are weaned off within 7 days from the first SBT. They constitute 15–20% of the patients. The last group constitutes those with a "prolonged weaning" who require more than 3 SBTs and more than 7 days from the first SBT for successful weaning.[2]

**Table 2: Parameters to Assess Spontaneous Breathing Trial Failure**

| Subjective indices | Objective parameters |
|---|---|
| • Agitation and anxiety | • $PaO_2$ <50–60 mmHg or $SaO_2$ <90% on $FiO_2$ >0.5 |
| • Depressed mental status | • $PaCO_2$ >50 mmHg or increase >8 mmHg |
| • Diaphoresis | • pH <7.32 or decrease by >0.07 |
| • Cyanosis | • RR >35 breath/min or increase >50% |
| • Evidence of increasing effort | • HR >140 breath/min or increase >20% |
| • Increased accessory muscle activity | • SBP >180 mmHg or increase >20% |
| • Facial signs of distress | • SBP <90 mmHg |
| • Dyspnea | • Cardiac arrhythmias |

RR, respiratory rate; HR, heart rate; SBP, systolic blood pressure.

## FAILURE OF SPONTANEOUS BREATHING TRIAL

Once the patient fails an SBT, various factors that could be causative should be looked into and possibly corrected[2] (Table 3).

In patients who fail the initial SBT, various modes of ventilation have been studied for early extubation. In a study comparing intermittent SBT, PSV, and

**Table 3: Common Considerations for Causes of Weaning Failure**

| | Pathophysiology | Possible causes |
|---|---|---|
| Respiratory load | • Increased work of breathing<br>• Reduced pulmonary compliance<br>• Increased resistive load | • Patient ventilator asynchrony<br>• Pneumonia, pulmonary edema<br>• Bronchospasm, retained secretions |
| Cardiac load | • Underlying cardiac dysfunction<br>• Change from positive to negative pressure ventilation | • Increased venous return<br>• Increased afterload |
| Neuromuscular competence | • Depressed central drive<br>• Peripheral dysfunction | • Poor $CO_2$ responsiveness,<br>• Sedatives, metabolic alkalosis<br>• Primary neuromuscular disorders<br>• Critical illness neuromuscular abnormality |
| Neuropsychological factors | • Delirium<br>• Anxiety/depression | • Drug induced, untreated pain, sleep deprivation |
| Metabolic disorders | • Hypophosphatemia<br>• Hypokalemia<br>• Hypomagnesemia | |
| Endocrine disorders | • Hypothyroidism<br>• Hypoadrenalism | |
| Ventilator-induced diaphragmatic dysfunction | • Diaphragmatic dysfunction due to assisted ventilation | |

synchronized intermittent mandatory ventilation (SIMV) as weaning modes for patients failing the initial SBT, lower numbers of weaning failures were found in the PSV group compared to the other two modes.[7] In another study comparing intermittent SBT, once a day SBT, PSV, and SIMV in a similar patient population, it was found that a once-daily trial of spontaneous breathing led to extubation about 3 times more quickly than intermittent mandatory ventilation and about twice as quickly as pressure-support ventilation. There was no significant difference in once-daily SBT as compared to intermittent SBT.[8]

## EXTUBATION

Once the patient tolerates an SBT, extubation is planned. Extubation constitutes an important step in critical care practice. Before extubation, there are several factors which need assessment. These include patient's ability to protect airway, quantity of secretions, sensorium, and strength of cough for airway clearance.

### Cuff Leak Test

Postextubation stridor or upper airway obstruction is known to occur due to various mechanisms in 2–16% of patients. These include glottis edema, prolonged intubation leading to inflammation of upper airways, and mucosal ulceration due to excessive cuff pressure.

To predict the above, cuff leak test (CLT) is advised before extubation. On volume-controlled ventilation (VCV) mode, a preset inspired VT and subsequent expired VT after cuff deflation are recorded. The difference tidal volume between VTi (inspired tidal volume) and average of 3 lowest VTe (expired tidal volume) is calculated. Leak of less than 110–130 mL (10–15.5%) is considered positive and indicates a high risk of postextubation stridor. The usual cut offs used are 110 mL and 15%. The test has a high specificity and negative predictive value (99% and 98% respectively) but a low sensitivity and positive predictive value (80%).[9]

The utility of steroids in such patients to reduce the incidence of postextubation stridor, though documented in studies is not yet well established and no standard protocol has been established. One suggested protocol includes treatment with 40 mg methylprednisolone 6 hourly for 24 hours before extubation.[10]

## POSTEXTUBATION PERIOD

The process of weaning does not end with extubation but also encompasses the postextubation period. Monitoring clinical parameters are of utmost importance in the postextubation period. Features that suggest postextubation failure and need for reintubation are depicted in table 4.

**Table 4: Parameters Suggesting Postextubation Failure**

- RR >25 breaths/min for 2 hours
- HR >140 beats/min or a sustained increase or decrease of >20%
- Clinical signs of respiratory muscle fatigue or increased work of breathing
- $SaO_2$ <90%; $PaO_2$ <80 mmHg on $FiO_2$ >0.50
- Hypercapnia ($PaCO_2$ >45 mmHg or >20% increase from pre-extubation), pH <7.33

RR, respiratory rate; HR, heart rate.

**Table 5: Risk Factors for Postextubation Failure**

- Elderly patients (age >65 years)
- More than one consecutive failure of weaning trial
- Chronic heart failure
- $PaCO_2$ >45 mmHg after extubation
- More than one medical/surgical comorbid illness
- Poor cough reflex
- Stridor at extubation that does not require immediate reintubation
- APACHE II score >12 on the day of extubation
- Severely obese patients (body mass index >35 $kg/m^2$)

APACHE II, Acute Physiology and Chronic Health Evaluation II.

There have been many risk factors associated with postextubation failure and these have been illustrated in table 5.[11]

Weaning success is defined as extubation and the absence of ventilatory support for 48 hours following the extubation. Failure of SBT or need for reintubation within 48 hours of extubation is considered weaning failure. For patients who are extubated but continued on ventilator support through noninvasive method the term "weaning in progress" is suggested.[2]

## PARAMETERS PREDICTING SPONTANEOUS BREATHING TRIAL OUTCOME

Various indices that can predict the probable outcome of a weaning trial have been studied. Some of these are readily available like minute ventilation, frequency/VT ratio. Some are integrated indices like CROP which incorporates compliance, RR, oxygenation ($PaO_2/PAO_2$), and maximum inspiratory pressure (PImax). None of these indices alone have been found to be sensitive and specific enough to be clinically useful in predicting the weaning outcome of an individual patient[12] (Table 6).

Most frequently used among these is the RSBI. It has been found to be the most accurate predictor of weaning outcome with sensitivity and specificity of 72–97% and 11–64%, respectively.[13] In a study comparing various predictive indices, RSBI was found to be the most accurate with the highest area under

| Table 6: Predictive Indexes for Weaning Outcome | |
| --- | --- |
| **Parameters** | **Threshold values** |
| Minute ventilation (Ve) | 10–15 L/min |
| PImax | –15 to –30 cm $H_2O$ |
| P0.1/PImax | <0.3 |
| CROP | 13 |
| RSBI (f/VT) | <60–105 min/L |

PImax, maximal insipiratory pressure; CROP, compliance, rate, oxygenation, pressure; RSBI, rapid shallow breathing index, VT, tidal volume.

curve (0.89).[14] Practically, it is easy to determine and does not require any special attachments in the ventilator.

## Maximal Inspiratory Pressure

Maximal inspiratory pressure (also called negative inspiratory force) is commonly used to test respiratory muscle strength and, in particular, the diaphragm. The proximal end of the endotracheal tube is occluded for 20–25 seconds with a one-way valve that allows the patient to exhale but not to inhale. This procedure leads to increasing inspiratory effort and PImax is measured toward the end of the occlusion period. PImax less than or equal to –20 to –30 cm $H_2O$ has a high sensitivity (ranging from 86 to 100%) and low specificity (ranging from 7 to 69%) for predicting successful liberation from mechanical ventilation.[1] It can be measured by incorporating a one-way valve in the breathing circuit.

## Airway Occlusion Pressure (P0.1)

Airway occlusion pressure is the pressure at the airway opening measured 0.1 seconds after inspiration against an occluded airway. It is effort independent and a good measure of respiratory drive. A threshold value of less than 4.5 cm $H_2O$ to less than 6 cm $H_2O$ has been shown to predict successful weaning. The ratio of P0.1 to PImax of less than 0.3 has been found to be a good predictor of weaning outcome and better than each of them used alone.[1,13]

Newer ventilators have in built modules to measure P0.1 and PImax without any need for special instrumentation.

## Compliance, Rate, Oxygenation, Pressure Index

It is an integrative index that incorporates respiratory system compliance (Crs), spontaneous breathing frequency (f), arterial to alveolar oxygenation ratio ($PaO_2/PAO_2$), and PImax.

$$CROP = [Crs \times PImax \times (PaO_2/PAO_2)]/f$$

A value of value greater than 13 mL/breaths/minute offers a reasonably accurate prediction of weaning outcome. But it carries the disadvantage of being complicated for bedside analysis.[1,13] It has a sensitivity of around 81% and a specificity of about 57% to predict successful weaning.

## NEWER MODES OF VENTILATION FOR WEANING

### Automatic Tube Compensation

The use of automatic tube compensation (ATC) aims at compensating for the nonlinear pressure drop across the endotracheal tube during spontaneous breathing. PSV may under-correct for the work of breathing early in the inspiratory phase and over-correct in the latter part during low flow. Addition of ATC to PSV can decrease the work of breathing by 30–50% compared to PSV alone. It has been found to be comparable to other modes of weaning in various studies.[15]

### Proportional Assist Ventilation

In simple terms in proportional assist ventilation (PAV), ventilator amplifies the inspiratory effort made by the patient. It has not been assessed systematically for weaning in trials.

### Adaptive Servo-ventilation (Computer-based Weaning)

Also known as "automated weaning", adaptive servo-ventilation (ASV) aims at rapid adaptation of ventilator support to the changing patient status. ASV recognizes spontaneous breathing and automatically switches between mandatory pressure-controlled breaths and spontaneous pressure-supported breaths in patients. If the spontaneous rate is less than the set target, it acts as SIMV and as PSV if spontaneous rate is greater. Compared to manual weaning, it has been found to reduce the duration of mechanical ventilation and length of ICU stay.[16] However, other studies have shown no significant difference compared to manual weaning.[17]

### Neurally Adjusted Ventilatory Assist

Neurally adjusted ventilatory assist (NAVA) is an assist mode of ventilation which delivers a pressure support proportional to the electrical activity of the diaphragm (EAdi). The level of support is therefore determined by the patient's respiratory center neural output. The diaphragmatic potentials are sensed by esophageal probe inserted as a nasogastric tube. Since the ventilator is triggered and cycled off based on the diaphragmatic potentials, NAVA is likely to reduce patient ventilator asynchrony, a major factor responsible for delayed weaning.[18]

## Noninvasive Ventilation in Weaning

Noninvasive ventilation (NIV) has secured a prominent role in the management of acute respiratory failure. It has been studied in three different ways for weaning:[19]

- As part of an early weaning strategy, when patient fails SBT
- After weaning and extubation to prevent postextubation failure
- For postextubation failure, to prevent reintubation.

In the first case in chronic obstructive pulmonary disease (COPD) patients, NIV was found to reduce the duration of mechanical ventilation, ICU stay, incidence of VAP and 60-day mortality in various studies.[20]

Preventive use of NIV postextubation has not shown any benefit in reducing extubation failure rate or mortality rate.[21] However, it has been recommended for patients at high risk of postextubation failure, i.e., age greater than 65 years, Acute Physiology and Chronic Health Evaluation II (APACHE II) greater than 12 at extubation, cardiac failure at intubation, and body mass index (BMI) greater than 35 kg/m$^2$.

In COPD patients who develop postextubation failure, NIV should be used cautiously.[4] It is not recommended for non-COPD patients with postextubation failure as a trend toward increased mortality due to delayed reintubations has been observed.[22]

## Role of Tracheostomy

A tracheostomy is commonly performed in the ICU whenever prolonged mechanical ventilation is anticipated in a critically ill patient. The possible benefits of tracheostomy that may facilitate weaning are reduced dead space, less airway resistance, improved patient comfort, less need for sedation, better glottic function, with less risk of aspiration, early weaning, and reduced incidence of VAP.[23] None of these have been have been proven consistently in studies. This is because of the extreme heterogeneity of the studies conducted thus far.

The optimal timing of tracheostomy has been unanswered till date. A meta-analysis including four trials showed that early tracheostomy (<7 vs. >7 days) reduced the duration of mechanical ventilation and the length of ICU stay with no significant effect on VAP and mortality.[24] However, a recent randomized trial failed to demonstrate any benefit of early over late tracheostomy (<4 vs. >10 days).[25]

## CONCLUSION

Weaning is a gradual process of liberation from mechanical ventilation and resumption of spontaneous breathing. Weaning process should start as early as possible, as delay in weaning leads to poor outcome. All patients should be assessed daily for readiness to wean. Daily sedation-free interval and spontaneous awakening trial helps in early weaning. Improving primary disease status, hemodynamic stability, metabolic parameters, sensorium, and adequate oxygenation are some important parameters to assess for weaning. Spontaneous breathing trial can be given by three ways: PSV, continuous positive airway pressure, or T-piece trial and all of them equal predictability for successful weaning. A 30-minute SBT is as good as 120-minute SBT. Cuff leak test and assessment for patient's ability to handle secretions should be done before removal of endotracheal tube. Elderly age, multiple comorbidities and morbid obesity are few of the factors that predict extubation failure. Various indices like PImax, P0.1, P0.1/PImax, and CROP index may be useful to predict successful weaning. Newer modes of ventilation like PAV, ASV, and NAVA may be useful for weaning especially in difficult weaning. An early tracheostomy probably helps in weaning though the issue of timing of tracheostomy remains controversial.

### Editor's Comment

*Weaning or liberating one from the ventilator is a science and art. Once a patient on a ventilator has stabilized, the next step is to get him or her off the ventilator. This process of weaning is started by assessing whether the patient is fit to be weaned off. Assessment for weaning should be considered as early as possible, as delays in getting the patient off the ventilator are associated with higher complications and increased mortality. Once the deemed patient is fit, various methods are used for a spontaneous breathing trial. These could be a continuous or intermittent T piece trial, using an intermittent mandatory ventilation mode or weaning with pressure support during the spontaneous breathing trial. None has comprehensively shown to be superior to the other and a simple T piece trial is usually sufficient. Once the patient is off the ventilator, the next step is to assess fitness for extubation. Many patients have a lot of secretions and a poor cough reflex. In those patients, although they are breathing spontaneously, the endotracheal tube is kept in place for airway management and clearing secretions. Many new methods, including neurally adjusted ventilatory assist, have been introduced to help the weaning process ventilation. However, it is unclear currently as to how helpful these processes are in facilitating early weaning.*

***Randeep Guleria***

## REFERENCES


1. El-Khatib MF, Bou-Khalil P. Clinical review: liberation from mechanical ventilation. *Crit Care.* 2008;12(4):221.
2. Boles JM, Bion J, Connors A, Herridge M, Marsh B, Melot C, et al. Weaning from mechanical ventilation. *Eur Respir J.* 2007;29(5):1033-56.
3. Kollef MH, Levy NT, Ahrens TS, Schaiff R, Prentice D, Sherman G. The use of continuous i.v. sedation is associated with prolongation of mechanical ventilation. *Chest.* 1998;114(2):541-8.
4. Kress JP, Pohlman AS, O'Connor MF, Hall JB. Daily interruption of sedative infusions in critically ill patients undergoing mechanical ventilation. *N Engl J Med.* 2000;342(20):1471-7.
5. Esteban A, Alía I, Gordo F, Fernández R, Solsona JF, Vallverdú I, et al. Extubation outcome after spontaneous breathing trials with T-tube or pressure support ventilation. The Spanish Lung Failure Collaborative Group. *Am J Respir Crit Care Med.* 1997;156:459-65.
6. Esteban A, Alía I, Tobin MJ, Gil A, Gordo F, Vallverdú I, et al. Effect of spontaneous breathing trial duration on outcome of attempts to discontinue mechanical ventilation. Spanish Lung Failure Collaborative Group. *Am J Respir Crit Care Med.* 1999;159(2):512-8.
7. Brochard L, Rauss A, Benito S, Conti G, Mancebo J, Rekik N, et al. Comparison of three methods of gradual withdrawal from ventilatory support during weaning from mechanical ventilation. *Am J Respir Crit Care Med.* 1994;150(4):896-903.
8. Esteban A, Frutos F, Tobin MJ, Alía I, Solsona JF, Valverdú I, et al. A comparison of four methods of weaning patients from mechanical ventilation. Spanish Lung Failure Collaborative Group. *N Engl J Med.* 1995;332(6):345-50.
9. Miller RL, Cole RP. Association between reduced cuff leak volume and postextubation stridor. *Chest.* 1996;110(4):1035-40.
10. Cheng KC, Hou CC, Huang HC, Lin SC, Zhang H. Intravenous injection of methylprednisolone reduces the incidence of postextubation stridor in intensive care unit patients. *Crit Care Med.* 2006;34(5):1345-50.
11. Agarwal R, Aggarwal AN, Gupta D, Jindal SK. Role of noninvasive positive-pressure ventilation in postextubation respiratory failure: a meta-analysis. *Respir Care.* 2007;52(11):1472-9.
12. MacIntyre N. Discontinuing mechanical ventilatory support. *Chest.* 2007;132(3):1049-56.
13. Manthous CA, Schmidt GA, Hall JB. Liberation from mechanical ventilation: a decade of progress. *Chest.* 1998;114(3):886-901.
14. Yang KL, Tobin MJ. A prospective study of indexes predicting the outcome of trials of weaning from mechanical ventilation. *N Engl J Med.* 1991;324(21):1445-50.
15. Haberthür C, Mols G, Elsasser S, Bingisser R, Stocker R, Guttmann J. Extubation after breathing trials with automatic tube compensation, T-tube, or pressure support ventilation. *Acta Anaesthesiol Scand.* 2002;46(8):973-9.
16. Lellouche F, Mancebo J, Jolliet P, Roeseler J, Schortgen F, Dojat M, et al. A multicenter randomized trial of computer-driven protocolized weaning from mechanical ventilation. *Am J Respir Crit Care Med.* 2006;174(8):894-900.
17. Taniguchi C, Eid RC, Saghabi C, Souza R, Silva E, Knobel E, et al. Automatic versus manual pressure support reduction in the weaning of post-operative patients: a randomised controlled trial. *Crit Care.* 2009;13(1):R6.
18. Terzi N, Piquilloud L, Rozé H, Mercat A, Lofaso F, Delisle S, et al. Clinical review: update on neurally adjusted ventilatory assist—report of a round-table conference. *Crit Care.* 2012;16(3):225.
19. Chawla R, Khilnani GC, Suri JC, Ramakrishnan N, Mani RK, Prayag S, et al. Guidelines for noninvasive ventilation in acute respiratory failure. *Indian J Crit Care Med.* 2006;10:117-47.
20. Ferrer M, Valencia M, Nicolas JM, Bernadich O, Badia JR, Torres A. Early noninvasive ventilation averts extubation failure in patients at risk: a randomized trial. *Am J Respir Crit Care Med.* 2006;173(2):164-70.
21. Su CL, Chiang LL, Yang SH, Lin HI, Cheng KC, Huang YC, et al. Preventive use of noninvasive ventilation after extubation: a prospective, multicenter randomized controlled trial. *Respir Care.* 2012;57(2):204-10.

22. Esteban A, Frutos-Vivar F, Ferguson ND, Arabi Y, Apezteguía C, González M, et al. Noninvasive positive-pressure ventilation for respiratory failure after extubation. *N Engl J Med*. 2004;350(24):2452-60.
23. Pierson DJ. Tracheostomy and weaning. *Respir Care*. 2005;50(4):526-33.
24. Griffiths J, Barber VS, Morgan L, Young JD. Systematic review and meta-analysis of studies of the timing of tracheostomy in adult patients undergoing artificial ventilation. *BMJ*. 2005;330(7502):1243.
25. Young D, Harrison DA, Cuthbertson BH, Rowan K; TracMan Collaborators. Effect of early vs. late tracheostomy placement on survival in patients receiving mechanical ventilation: the TracMan randomized trial. *JAMA*. 2013;309(20):2121-9.

World Clin Pulm Crit Care Med. 2016;4(1):48-65.

# Management of Acute Severe Chronic Obstructive Pulmonary Disease and Asthma

[1,*]Rajesh Chawla MD FCCP FCCM,
[2]Deven Juneja DNB FNB EDIC FCCP IFCCM FCCM

[1]Department of Respiratory Medicine, Critical Care and Sleep Medicine, Indraprastha Apollo Hospitals
New Delhi, India
[2]Department of Critical Care and Emergency Medicine, Shri Balaji Action Medical Institute
New Delhi, India

## ABSTRACT

Diseases of chronic airflow limitation like chronic obstructive pulmonary disease and asthma are the leading causes of morbidity and mortality worldwide. These patients require frequent hospitalizations because of their acute decompensation and a significant proportion of these patients require intensive care unit care. These exacerbations have a profound effect on the pulmonary function and quality of life in these patients apart from tremendous financial implications. Apart from early aggressive care with bronchodilators, a selective subgroup of patients may require treatment with steroids and antibiotics. A significant proportion of these patients may also require ventilatory support which may be invasive or noninvasive. Hence, the physicians should be able to recognize the crisis early to take appropriate steps for better patient outcomes.

## INTRODUCTION

Diseases of chronic airflow limitation like chronic obstructive pulmonary disease (COPD) and asthma are the leading causes of morbidity and mortality worldwide.[1] COPD is one of the leading causes of death and it is predicted that the rate with which the incidence of this disease is increasing, it is soon going to be the third leading cause of mortality and the fifth cause of burden of disease, worldwide.[1-3] Like COPD, an increasing number of people are affected with asthma, with the

---

*Corresponding author
*Email:* drchawla@hotmail.com

current estimates suggesting that around 150 million people are suffering from this disease globally. In India alone, there are an estimated 20 million asthmatics.[4] Even though the morbidity associated with the disease is much more than the associated mortality, the annual reported death rate is 180,000.

The underlying pathophysiology in asthma includes inflammation, hyperresponsiveness, and remodeling of airways resulting in airflow obstruction which is completely reversible either spontaneously or with therapy. However, if asthma is not treated appropriately or there is recurrent obstruction, the airflow obstruction can become permanent due to alteration of the bronchial mucosa and then these patients may clinically present like COPD. So differentiation between COPD and asthma may be challenging, especially in smokers and older asthmatics. In a significant proportion of patients, clinical features of both COPD and asthma may coexist. This clinical condition is well recognized now and is labeled as asthma-COPD overlap syndrome (ACOS).[5]

Asthma flare-up (exacerbation) is an acute or subacute worsening in symptoms and lung functions from the patient's usual status; occasionally it may be initial presentation of asthma.

An acute exacerbation of COPD may be defined as an acute episode which is characterized clinically by worsening of the patient's respiratory symptoms or signs which is beyond normal day-to-day variations and requires a change in the medications. These exacerbations may range in severity from mild or transient decrease in functional status to fatal events. Each exacerbation may lead to reduction in lung function and quality of life and may be associated with an increased risk of death.[6,7]

Different subsets of asthma have been described.[8-10] "Severe asthma" is a vital subset of asthma affecting 5–10% of asthmatics, generally defined as a disease not responsive to ongoing therapy, including systemic steroids.[8]

These patients of COPD and asthma with chronic airway diseases require frequent hospitalizations because of their acute decompensation and a significant proportion of these patients require intensive care unit (ICU) care.[3] As a result, these exacerbations may cause a significant economic and social burden on the healthcare resources. In terms of financial burden, COPD presently is a more costly disease compared to asthma because of its high incidence and greater morbidity. Because of profound effect of these exacerbations, their prevention and treatment is now recognized as the primary goal of COPD management.[11]

## CAUSES OF ACUTE SEVERE CHRONIC OBSTRUCTIVE PULMONARY DISEASE AND ASTHMA

Most important cause of exacerbations in patients with COPD is infections, which may be bacterial, viral, or fungal. Infections are responsible for more than

50% of the exacerbations. Other causes include air pollutants or tobacco smoke, seasonal changes, and poor compliance to therapy.[11,12]

Common bacterial pathogens causing exacerbation in COPD include *Streptococcus pneumoniae, Haemophilus influenzae, Moraxella catarrhalis,* and *Enterobacteriaceae spp.* Patients with severe disease or those who require frequent hospitalizations may be at a risk of developing *Pseudomonas aeruginosa* infection. On the other hand, *Rhinovirus spp* and influenza virus are commonly implicated viral agents.

On the other side, acute severe asthma is generally not associated with any bacterial infections and causes include noncompliance with therapy, exposure to allergens, pollution or tobacco smoke, and use of drugs like nonsteroidal anti-inflammatory drugs (NSAIDs) or β-blockers.[13] Infections, if present, are mostly viral in etiology.[14]

## CLINICAL PRESENTATION

Acute severe asthma and COPD usually present with sudden increase in symptoms like acute worsening breathlessness cough, sputum production, chest tightness, and wheezing. Other associated symptoms include fever, chest pain, increased tiredness, and increase in oxygen requirement.[15] History of poorly controlled asthma in the recent past is a major risk factor for acute severe asthma.

There are certain other differential diagnoses which must be considered when evaluating these patients (Table 1).

## ASSESSMENT OF SEVERITY

Several clinical elements must be considered when evaluating patients with exacerbations. These include the severity of the underlying disease, presence of comorbidities, and history of previous exacerbations with their severity. The physical examination should evaluate effect of an episode on the hemodynamic parameters and respiratory system.

The initial patient management includes detailed history taking and a thorough clinical examination. Every effort should be made to illicit the potential cause of

| Table 1: Differential Diagnosis of Acute Exacerbation of Asthma and Chronic Obstructive Pulmonary Disease | |
|---|---|
| • Congestive heart failure | • Bronchiolitis obliterans |
| • Pulmonary embolism | • Pneumothorax |
| • Bronchiectasis | • Diffuse panbronchiolitis |
| • Respiratory tract infections | • Mechanical airway obstruction |

exacerbation, assess the severity of illness, and associated organ dysfunction. Close monitoring of patients is essential as early detection of trend toward improvement or deterioration is of paramount importance, especially in patients with asthma.

Presence of certain clinical signs suggests worsening acute severe asthma (Table 2). These include tachypnea, tachycardia, and reduced peak expiratory flow rate (PEFR) less than 40% of the expected normal or best normal value.[16] As the severity progresses, they may not be able to complete sentences or lie down flat. Patient may be in respiratory distress using accessory muscles of respiration.

Signs like inability to maintain respiratory effort or silent chest on auscultation, presence of cyanosis, confusion or coma, bradycardia, hypotension, or nonquantifiable PEFR suggest life-threatening situation.

Pulmonary function tests are useful in diagnosing asthma and COPD, assessing their severity and following the progress of the disease. However, its utility is limited in patients with exacerbation.

In patients with asthma, serial monitoring of lung function by measuring PEFR or forced expiratory volume in 1 second (FEV1) at bedside is vitally important and they can be used to estimate the severity of an attack. A PEFR or FEV1 value lesser than 30–50% of predicted or personal best signifies a severe attack. In addition, lack of improvement in PEFR or FEV1, even after aggressive medical therapy predicts a more severe course of asthma.[17] However, it is generally not recommended to measure PEFR or FEV1 when the patient is having a severe attack, as the deep inspiration maneuver required in their measurement may worsen bronchospasm precipitating a respiratory arrest.[18] For COPD patient, spirometry during acute exacerbation is not recommended.

In addition to clinical assessment, arterial blood gas (ABG) analysis is also the best marker to assess the acuteness and severity of the exacerbation. In patients with COPD, any pH below 7.3 with high $CO_2$ level signifies acute decompensation. On the other hand, in patients with asthma, even a mild increase in $CO_2$ level with fall in pH signifies severe disease and fatigue. Serial monitoring of ABGs should be done for arterial oxygen tension ($PaO_2$), arterial $CO_2$ tension ($PaCO_2$), and pH which may aid in assessing the response to therapy and to detect any deterioration in clinical condition.

**Table 2: Features of Acute Severe Exacerbation of Asthma**

- Increase in dyspnea
- Patient unable to complete one sentence in one breath
- Tachypnea (respiratory rate >30/minute)
- Tachycardia (heart rate >120/minute)
- Use of accessory muscles of respiration
- Pulsus paradoxus (>25 mmHg fall in systolic blood pressure on inspiration)
- Peak expiratory flow <40% personal best or <200 L/minute

The oxygen saturation ($SpO_2$) can be monitored using pulse oximetry and is useful for trending and adjusting oxygen levels. The goals of oxygen therapy in patients of COPD are to maintain a $PaO_2$ level above 60 mmHg and $SpO_2$ level around 90%. These levels will prevent tissue hypoxia and preserve cellular oxygenation. Because of the shape of the oxyhemoglobin dissociation curve, increasing the $PaO_2$ levels much higher than 60 mmHg has little added benefit but may increase the chances of $CO_2$ retention in COPD patients, thereby causing respiratory acidosis.

## ADDITIONAL INVESTIGATIONS

Investigations may not be required to make a diagnosis of exacerbation, but they may aid in assessment of severity, planning the appropriate therapy, and assessing the response to therapy. Routine investigations like complete blood count, renal function tests, and electrolytes should be done for all patients.

Electrolyte abnormalities are common in these patients. COPD patients have a tendency to retain sodium. Hypokalemia is also common in these patients due to intake of drugs like β-adrenergic agonists, steroids, and diuretics. β-adrenergic agonists may also lead to hypocalcemia and hypomagnesemia due to their increased renal excretion. COPD patients with chronic respiratory acidosis develop compensatory metabolic alkalosis and hence serum bicarbonate levels may be useful in assessing disease progression.

A chest X-ray should be done in all patients which may be helpful in identifying the cause of exacerbation, detecting any associated complications, and to rule out other differential diagnosis.

Computed tomography (CT) chest is rarely indicated in ICU patients. It may be done in patients refractory to therapy, to rule out any associated complications or when the diagnosis is in doubt.

Electrocardiogram (ECG) and echocardiogram may be required to rule out any cardiac abnormality and to assess cardiac status if features of cor pulmonale are present.

Cultures should not be routinely sent in all patients. In patients having purulent sputum, it should be sent for Gram stain and aerobic culture. As Gram stain report may become available in a few hours, it may aid in identifying the organism and aid in initial antibiotic therapy. Blood cultures should be obtained if the patient has a history of fever.

### Biomarkers

Biomarkers for severe COPD and asthma have been obtained from biofluids, tissue, and exhaled breath samples. Even though several biomarkers have been studied extensively, no biomarker has been found to be reliable in differentiating COPD from asthma.[19,20]

Among the various biomarkers, sputum eosinophil levels and exhaled nitric oxide levels have been the most widely studied and established biomarkers in patients with asthma. These biomarkers have been found useful in determining disease activity and also response to anti-inflammatory therapy.[21] Exhaled nitric oxide has also been shown to be useful in predicting steroid responsiveness.[22]

Serum C-reactive protein (CRP) levels have been found to be elevated in patients with COPD, in whom it has been shown to predict risk of hospitalization and death.[21] 8-isoprostane is another oxidant marker that has been shown to be useful in patients with COPD exacerbation.[23] Other biomarkers which have been extensively studied in COPD patients include inflammatory plasma biomarkers, like fibrinogen, surfactant protein D and club cell secretory protein-16, which can help in identifying patients at risk of developing exacerbations and those who might have a more severe disease course.[22] However, we are still in pursuit to identify an ideal biomarker for patients with acute asthma and COPD.

## TREATMENT

The main aim of the treatment is to rapidly reduce the airflow obstruction and inflammation with help of bronchodilators and glucocorticoids, respectively (Table 3).

For management purposes, exacerbations of COPD have been simply classified as levels I, II, and III. Level I can be managed at home, level II requires hospitalization, and level III leads to respiratory failure and hence should be managed in ICUs.[26]

## Bronchodilators

Bronchodilators form the mainstay of therapy as they can rapidly cause bronchial smooth muscle relaxation.[27] Short-acting inhaled β2-agonist drugs like salbutamol inhaler/levosalbutamol with/without ipratropium bromide with spacer or nebulizer, as needed, should be initiated (Table 3). Inhalational therapy with metered-dose inhaler (MDI) or nebulizers are preferred over oral or intravenous routes because of improved efficacy. If the patient is hypercapnic, the nebulizer should be driven by compressed air, not oxygen, to avoid risk of worsening hypercapnia. If $SpO_2$ is low, oxygen can be administered simultaneously through nasal cannulae.

Side effects of β-agonists are rare and generally occur when high doses are given. These include tachycardia, tremors, hypokalemia and hyperglycemia. Long-acting β-agonists are not generally used in these acute cases.

| Table 3: Pharmacologic Management in Exacerbation of Asthma[13,16,24,25] | |
|---|---|
| **Agent** | **Dose** |
| β-agonists | • Inhaled β-agonists: Salbutamol 2.5–5 mg in 2.5 mL normal saline by nebulization every 20 minutes for three doses and then every 1–4 hours as needed or 4–8 puffs by metered-dose inhaler (MDI) with spacer every 20 minutes for three doses and then every 1–4 hours as needed<br>• Alternatively, in severe attack 10–15 mg can be administered by continuous nebulization |
| Anticholinergics | • Ipratropium bromide 0.5 mg by nebulization every 20 minutes for three doses or 4–8 puffs by MDI with spacer every 20 minutes as needed for up to 3 hours<br>• Ipratropium bromide can also be given combined with salbutamol |
| Corticosteroids | • Intravenous methylprednisolone 60–125 mg<br>• Intravenous hydrocortisone 100 mg<br>• Oral prednisone 40 mg |
| Methylxanthines | • Theophylline 5 mg/kg (intravenous) over 30 minutes—loading dose in patients not already on theophylline, followed by 0.4 mg/kg/hour intravenous maintenance dose. Serum levels should be checked within 6 hours |
| Additional treatment for asthma | • Adrenaline 0.3–0.4 mg of a 1:1,000 solution subcutaneously every 20 minutes for three doses<br>• Terbutaline subcutaneously (0.25 mg) or as intravenous infusion starting at 0.05–0.10 µg/kg/minute<br>• Magnesium sulfate 2 g over 20 minutes intravenously |

Inhaled anticholinergic agents like ipratropium are generally recommended in the management of exacerbations of COPD. However, several studies have shown that the combination of inhaled anticholinergics with β-agonists may be used in acute asthma patients with severe airflow obstruction as this combination results in a better bronchodilation than either drug used alone.[28-30] Hence, it is now recommended to be used in patients with acute severe asthma in emergency.[24]

## Systemic Corticosteroids

Oral or intravenous corticosteroids may also be considered if there are no significant contraindications. Steroids should be given for 7–14 days only. Oral prednisolone 40 mg daily or an equivalent dose of intravenous hydrocortisone, methylprednisolone, or dexamethasone may be initiated.

The primary aim of using steroids is to aid in reducing inflammation. It may not be useful in providing immediate clinical relief as it may take a few hours to have its effect. Hence, for the rapid symptomatic relief, inhaled short-acting β-agonist and anticholinergic drugs are vital. However, for a more long-term recovery, systemic steroids are useful.[24]

High-dose inhaled steroids are recommended for gradually worsening asthma but they are not recommended as an alternative to systemic steroids in acute severe asthma.

## Theophylline and Other Methylxanthines

Intravenous theophylline/aminophylline does not form the first line of therapy and their use is generally controversial and hence should be used only as an adjunct to nebulized bronchodilators, if adequate response is not achieved with bronchodilators alone. Caution should be exerted especially if the patient was already on oral theophylline, as it may increase the risk of toxicity. In addition, several drugs like phenytoin, ciprofloxacin, clarithromycin, allopurinol, etc. may have drug interactions and hence care must be exerted, when they are used with theophylline.

## Antibiotics

Antibiotics are not indicated in all patients with exacerbations of COPD and asthma. As exacerbations of asthma are generally not infective or are associated with viral infections only, the role of antibiotics is even less in such patients.

They are used more often in exacerbation of COPD. Antibiotics should be started only in patients producing purulent sputum. Antibiotics are also indicated if there is any change in color, consistency, or volume of sputum. If there is no change in sputum characteristics, antibiotics may be indicated in patients with clinical symptoms of pneumonia or in those with signs suggestive of pneumonia on chest radiograph. The choice of antibiotics should be based on the local resistance patterns, if available. Antibiotics must be changed accordingly, once culture sensitivity results become available. Antibiotics may be given for 7–10 days.

## Oxygen Therapy

Oxygen therapy is indicated in all patients with exacerbations to prevent tissue hypoxia with the goal of maintaining arterial oxygen saturation ($SaO_2$) at greater than 90%. Even though prevention of tissue hypoxia supersedes $CO_2$ retention issue, careful monitoring of clinical condition of the patient along with ABG and pulse oximetry is required.[31] Retention of $CO_2$ is generally not an issue in patients with asthma, hence they can be safely given higher oxygen concentration in the initial phase.

## Magnesium Sulfate

In asthmatic patients with refractory bronchospasm symptoms not resolving even after 1 hour of aggressive therapy, other drugs have been tried.[24] Magnesium sulfate, 2 g to be given over 20 minutes, may be used because of its bronchodilatory effects.[32]

## Other Therapies

Several other therapies have been tried in patients with refractory severe asthma. However, their role is controversial and they are generally not recommended. These include inhalational anesthetic agents, heliox and nitric oxide.

Inhalational anesthetic agents like halothane, isoflurane, and sevoflurane are potent bronchodilators and have been tried in asthmatic patients receiving mechanical ventilation and not responding to conventional therapies.[33] Heliox, a mixture of helium and oxygen has been shown to reduce the work of breathing and improve gas exchange due to its low density. However, it may reduce the concentration of inspired oxygen and its clinical efficacy is marginal.[34] Similarly, nitric oxide has been shown to have some bronchodilatory effect. In addition, it also dilates pulmonary arteries and may be useful in improving ventilation/ perfusion matching.[35]

# MECHANICAL VENTILATION

## Noninvasive Mechanical Ventilation

Pathophysiologically, these patients have high airway resistance, pulmonary hyperinflation, and increased pulmonary dead space. All these changes lead to increased work of breathing. The primary aim of mechanical ventilation in these patients is to improve gas exchange and to unload the compromised respiratory muscles so that they can recover from their fatigued state.

The recent years have witnessed increased use of noninvasive ventilation (NIV) in the management of patients with acute respiratory failure. This is mainly attributable to the advent of more comfortable and user-friendly interface and the improved awareness and accessibility of NIV in the recent years.[36-39]

Several studies have shown the efficacy of use of NIV in the management of COPD with reduced need for endotracheal intubation.[40-51] NIV has also been shown to be instrumental in reducing the length of ICU and hospital stay, incidence of nosocomial infections, and overall mortality.[41-43] Another advantage of NIV is that it can also be initiated outside ICU settings. However, patients with severe exacerbation (pH <7.30) should better be managed in the ICU setting. However, for maximal benefit, it should be initiated early, preferably before development of severe hypercapnia and respiratory acidosis. The benefits of NIV are less marked in patients with mild exacerbation.[52]

Most of the patients with COPD exacerbation may be safely and successfully managed with NIV. Hence, it is recommended that NIV should be considered in all patients with acute exacerbation of COPD (pH <7.35, $PaCO_2$ >45 mmHg) along with standard medical therapy.

The role of NIV in the management of acute exacerbation of asthma is less well defined even though several studies have shown that the use of NIV in such patients may improve lung functions, and improve symptoms faster.[53-56] Hence, NIV is not presently recommended in all patients with acute exacerbation of asthma but it may be tried in patients with severe acute asthma, not responding adequately to medical measures.[57,58] NIV in asthma should be initiated in an ICU where continuous monitoring and facilities for immediate endotracheal intubation are readily available.[58]

Noninvasive ventilation is also indicated in weaning the COPD patients from mechanical ventilation to prevent reintubation and atelectasis.[58]

Noninvasive ventilation should be avoided in the following patient populations:[59,60]

- Patients unable to protect their airways, like those with altered mental status
- Patients producing copious secretions
- Active gastrointestinal bleed
- Severe gastrointestinal symptoms like vomiting, obstructed bowel, gastro-intestinal surgery
- Hemodynamically unstable patients, those with uncontrolled arrhythmias, on high inotropic support, or with recent myocardial infarction.

Noninvasive ventilation can be applied using portable pressure ventilators or ICU ventilators. Portable pressure ventilators are commonly used in COPD patients. Initially, inspiratory positive airway pressure can be set at 8–10 cm $H_2O$ and expiratory positive airway pressures at 4–5 cm $H_2O$. The pressures can be increased gradually as per the patient's response, ensuring patient comfort, and ventilator synchrony.[58]

Close monitoring is required when patients are initiated on NIV, especially in the first few hours, and close watch on vital signs, sensorium and $SpO_2$, must be kept. ABG should be done at the end of 1–4 hours, to assess the response on NIV.[58]

Noninvasive ventilation should be applied for as long as possible in the initial 24 hours, thereafter, its duration can be reduced as per the patient's response.[58] Determinants of failure for NIV are given the table 4. NIV should be discontinued early in patients who are intolerant or unable to accept this therapy and in such patients low threshold should be kept for invasive mechanical ventilation (IMV).

| Table 4: Determinants of Failure for Noninvasive Ventilation in the Acute Setting |
|---|
| • Patient unable to coordinate with the noninvasive ventilation |
| • Persistent tachypnea |
| • Edentulous patient |
| • Persistent hypercapnia or respiratory acidosis |
| • High severity of illness (high APACHE score) |
| • Underlying severe lung infection |
| • Significant air leak |
| • Ph <7.10 |
| • Copious secretions |
| • $PaCO_2$ >90 mmHg |
| • Poor initial response |
| • Poor neurologic status |
| • Poor compliance |

APACHE, Acute Physiology and Chronic Health Evaluation.

## Invasive Mechanical Ventilation

In spite of all aggressive measures, standard medical therapy, and NIV support, a significant proportion of patients with acute exacerbation of COPD and asthma may require IMV. There are no well-defined criteria for initiation for IMV in patients of COPD. Broadly, indications for the application of IMV in COPD are given in the table 5.

In COPD patients, it is generally advocated that the patient should be intubated if there is no improvement after 1–4 hours of NIV trial as evidenced by clinical condition and blood gas analysis. In patients with exacerbation of asthma, even lower threshold should be kept for intubation after a NIV trial as the main goal of IMV is to maintain oxygenation and prevent respiratory arrest.

This decision to intubate in asthma is usually clinical based on serial clinical evaluations that include degree of respiratory difficulty (respiratory rate more than 40/minute, inability to complete sentences), severity of airflow limitation (degree of respiratory difficulty, PEFR), clinical features (use of accessory muscles, fatigue, altered sensorium), oxygenation, $CO_2$ level, and response to therapy. In bronchial asthma in the presence of decreased mental status and exhaustion, a $PaCO_2$ of 42 mmHg although technically normal may be a sign of severe respiratory failure requiring intubation. When the physician feels respiratory failure is progressing in spite of pharmacotherapy and is unlikely to reverse, intubation should be performed immediately before it becomes emergent when patient develops respiratory arrest.

At the time of intubation, endotracheal tube with the largest possible diameter should be used in order to reduce the resistance and facilitate clearance of secretions. It should be rapid sequence intubation. The oral route for intubation is preferred over the nasal route as it not only allows passage of an 8 mm or more

**Table 5: Indications for Initiation of Invasive Mechanical Ventilation in Chronic Obstructive Pulmonary Disease**

- Noninvasive positive pressure ventilation failure in chronic obstructive pulmonary disease: worsening of arterial blood gas (ABG) and/or pH in 1–4 hours; lack of improvement in ABGs and/or pH after 4 hours
- Severe respiratory acidosis (pH <7.2) with hypercapnia ($PaCO_2$ >60 mmHg)
- Life-threatening hypoxemia
- Persistent tachypnea >35 breaths/minute
- Altered mental status
- Sever acute respiratory failure with contraindications to use of noninvasive ventilation

size endotracheal tube but also decrease the incidence of ventilator-associated pneumonia.

Effective sedation may be indicated to prepare the patient for intubation and also to improve patient-ventilator synchrony. Moreover, effective sedation may be useful in reducing work of breathing and oxygen consumption, improve patient comfort, and reduce risk of barotrauma by avoiding high inspiratory pressures.[61,62] Hence, sedation may be useful in the initial 24–48 hours period. Drugs generally used for this purpose include midazolam, fentanyl, ketamine, and propofol. Ketamine and propofol are preferred as they also have bronchodilatory properties. One must remember that ketamine may raise blood pressure and intracranial pressures and propofol may cause hypotension.[61,63] Paralytic agents are rarely indicated when sedative agents are ineffective in providing patient-ventilator synchrony. When used, they should be withdrawn as early as possible, preferably within 48 hours period.

Invasive mechanical ventilation may be particularly challenging in patients with obstructive airway diseases due to airflow obstruction and air trapping. Because of prolonged expiration due to constricted airways, these patients are prone to develop auto-positive end-expiratory pressure (auto-PEEP) and dynamic hyperinflation which may lead to increased pulmonary pressures, barotrauma, worsening hypercapnia, and reduced blood return to right heart. The initial ventilator settings are given in the table 6.

The following measures may be done to reduce development of auto-PEEP:[67]

- Increase inspiratory flow rate to reduce the inspiratory time and hence increase the expiratory time
- Reduce the respiratory rate, in order to allow the inhaled gas time to be exhaled by prolonging the expiratory time
- Reduce the tidal volume, allowing reduced gas to be exhaled easily.

The goal should be to wean off the patient as early as possible after adequate time has elapsed to rest the respiratory muscles and to allow other medical treatment to have its effect on disease resolution.

<table>
<tr><td>Table 6: Initial Ventilator Settings[64-66]</td></tr>
<tr><td>

- Mode: controlled mode volume or pressure controlled
- $FiO_2$: 1.0
- Long expiratory time: I:E ratio >1:2
- Low tidal volume: 5–7 mL/kg
- Low ventilator rate: 8–10 breaths/minute
- Minute ventilation: 8–10 L/minute
- Inspiratory pressure: 30–35 cm $H_2O$ on pressure control ventilation
- Limit peak inspiratory pressure: to <40 cm $H_2O$
- Low positive end-expiratory pressure: 5 cm $H_2O$

</td></tr>
</table>

## Intensive Care Unit Management

Due to ambiguity in data related to outcomes of COPD patients admitted to ICU, there may be reluctance on part of physicians to admit such patients in ICU. However, studies have shown that short- and intermediate-term outcome of these patients is comparable to other cohorts of patients even though the long-term mortality remains high.[68-70] Moreover, the outcome of these patients may not be reliably predicted based on the premorbid factors like age, functional status, and pulmonary function tests and hence should not influence ones decision of admitting the patients to ICU.[68,69] The severity of respiratory dysfunction should dictate the need for ICU. Indications for ICU admission are given in the table 7.

Patients with asthma require ICU admission less often.[71] In addition, the recent years have witnessed a significant reduction in mortality rates associated acute exacerbation of asthma. This may largely be attributed to early diagnosis, aggressive medical management including steroids, and advances in mechanical ventilation.[72] The reported mortality associated with acute severe asthma is around 10%.[73,74]

Apart from the general severity assessment scores, several disease-specific prognostic scores have been developed and tried in patients with severe asthma

<table>
<tr><td>Table 7: Indications for Intensive Care Unit Admission</td></tr>
<tr><td>

- Impending or actual respiratory failure
- Inability to maintain oxygen saturation more than 90% in spite of high-flow oxygen therapy
- Presence of other end-organ dysfunction including renal, liver, or neurological dysfunction
- Hemodynamic instability
- Failure to respond to noninvasive ventilation trial
- Presence of increased signs of infection (pyrexia, increased sputum purulence/volume, etc.)
- Significant abnormalities on chest X-ray
- Clinical deterioration
- Patients requiring invasive mechanical ventilation

</td></tr>
</table>

**Table 8: Prognostic Markers in Intensive Care Unit**

- Age
- Prior functional status
- Body mass index
- Need for home oxygen
- Underlying comorbidities
- Baseline lung function
- Previous intensive care unit admissions
- Low Glasgow coma scale
- Cardiorespiratory arrest prior to ICU admission
- Length of hospital stay prior to ICU admission
- Severity of illness (as determined by high admission APACHE II score)
- Presence of cardiac dysrhythmias

ICU, intensive care unit; APACHE II, Acute Physiology and Chronic Health Evaluation II.

and COPD to predict the outcomes.[75,76] Several prognostic indicators have been studied, which may aid in determining outcomes of COPD and asthma patients admitted in ICUs (Table 8).[77,78]

## CONCLUSION

Patients with exacerbations of COPD and asthma may require frequent hospitalizations and ICU care. These exacerbations have a profound effect on the pulmonary function and quality of life in these patients apart from tremendous financial implications. Hence, the physicians should be able to recognize the crisis early to take appropriate steps for better patient outcomes. Medical management involves oxygen, inhaled bronchodilators, anticholinergics, steroids, and antibiotics. Inhalational therapy with MDI or nebulizers are preferred over oral or intravenous routes because of improved efficacy. Short-acting inhaled β2-agonist drugs like salbutamol inhaler/levosalbutamol with/without ipratropium bromide with spacer or nebulizer, as needed, are usually the first line of therapy. Many other agents have been tried but without significant success. A significant proportion of these patients may also require ventilator support. NIV support has been shown to prevent complications, shorten length of stay and improve outcomes, especially in COPD patients. Hence, a trial of NIV must be initiated in patients with acute exacerbations if no contraindication exists. Invasive mechanical ventilation may be particularly challenging in patients with obstructive airway diseases due to airflow obstruction and air trapping. This decision to intubate in asthma is usually clinical based on serial clinical evaluations that include degree of respiratory difficulty, severity of airflow limitation, clinical features, oxygenation, $CO_2$, level and response to therapy. Because of prolonged expiration due to constricted airways, these patients are prone to develop auto-PEEP and dynamic hyperinflation which may lead to increased pulmonary pressures, barotrauma, worsening hypercapnia, and reduced blood return to right heart. Ventilatory strategy includes high inspiratory flow rates, low tidal volume, and low respiratory rate to reduce the development of auto-PEEP. Apart from the general severity assessment scores, several disease-specific prognostic scores have been developed and tried in patients with severe asthma and COPD to predict the outcomes.[75,76] These prognostic indicators may aid in determining outcomes of COPD and asthma patients admitted in ICUs.

---

### Editor's Comment

*Although the number of cases with very severe asthma requiring ventilation has come down, the number of cases of severe chronic obstructive pulmonary disease (COPD) requiring both noninvasive and invasive ventilation has significantly increased over the last decade. In severe asthma the disease has progressed, asthma control is poor, and there is a need to step up therapy to maximum doses and consider novel therapies like anti–immunoglobulin E drugs, etc. Similarly, in severe COPD, one needs to optimize treatment and explore even nonpharmacological options. It is also crucial to be able to objectively assess the patient to see if he or she is responding or worsening so that timely interventions can be done. Simple bedside measurement of vital signs and looking at pulse oximetry are helpful. With good medications and supportive care, the mortality in acute severe COPD and asthma has substantially improved over the years.*

***Randeep Guleria***

---

## REFERENCES


1. Mannino DM, Homa DM, Akinbami LJ, Ford ES, Redd SC. Chronic obstructive pulmonary disease surveillance—United States, 1971–2000. *MMWR Surveill Summ.* 2002;51:1-16.
2. Mackay AJ, Hurst JR. COPD exacerbations: causes, prevention, and treatment. *Immunol Allergy Clin North Am.* 2013;33:95-115.
3. Stoller JK. Clinical practice. Acute exacerbations of chronic obstructive pulmonary disease. *N Engl J Med.* 2002;346:988-94.
4. WHO Fact sheets. [online] Available from: http://www.who.int/mediacentre/factsheets/fs206/en/. [Accessed July, 2015].
5. Nakawah MO, Hawkins C, Barbandi F. Asthma, chronic obstructive pulmonary disease (COPD), and the overlap syndrome. *J Am Board Fam Med.* 2013;26(4):470-7.
6. Aaron SD, Vandemheen KL, Clinch JJ, Ahuja J, Brison RJ, Dickinson G, et al. Measurement of short-term changes in dyspnea and disease-specific quality of life following an acute COPD exacerbation. *Chest.* 2002;121(3):688-96.
7. Seemungal TA, Donaldson GC, Paul EA, Bestall JC, Jeffries DJ, Wedzicha JA. Effect of exacerbation on quality of life in patients with chronic obstructive pulmonary disease. *Am J Respir Crit Care Med.* 1998;157(5 Pt 1):1418-22.

8. Busse WW, Banks-Schlegel S, Wenzel SE. Pathophysiology of severe asthma. *J Allergy Clin Immunol.* 2000;106:1033-42.

9. Barnes PJ, Woolcock AJ. Difficult asthma. *Eur Respir J.* 1998;12:1208-18.

10. Ayres JG, Miles JF, Barnes PJ. Brittle asthma. *Thorax.* 1998;58:315-21.

11. Global initiative for chronic obstructive lung disease (GOLD). Global strategy for the diagnosis, management, and prevention of COPD. (2015). [online] Available from www.goldcopd.org/guidelines-global-strategy-for-diagnosis-management.html. [Accessed July, 2015].

12. Garcia-Aymerich J, Monso E, Marrades RM, Escarrabill J, Félez MA, Sunyer J, et al. Risk factors for hospitalization for a chronic obstructive pulmonary disease exacerbation. *Am J Respir Crit Care Med.* 2001;164:1002-7.

13. Jindal SK, Gupta D, Aggarwal AN, Agarwal R; World Health Organization; Government of India. Guidelines for management of asthma at primary and secondary levels of health care in India (2005). Indian J Chest Dis Allied Sci. 2005;47:309-43.

14. Corne JM, Marshall C, Smith S, Schreiber J, Sanderson G, Holgate ST, et al. Frequency, severity, and duration of rhinovirus infections in asthmatic and non-asthmatic individuals: a longitudinal cohort study. *Lancet.* 2002;359:831-4.

15. Anthonisen NR, Manfreda J, Warren CP, Hershfield ES, Harding GK, Nelson NA. Antibiotic therapy in exacerbations of chronic obstructive pulmonary disease. *Ann Intern Med.* 1987;106(2):196-204.

16. Rai SP, Patil SP, Vardhan V, Marwah V, Pethe M, Pandey IM. Best treatment guidelines for bronchial asthma. *MJAFI.* 2007;63:264-8.

17. Rodrigo G, Rodrigo C. Assessment of the patient with acute asthma in the emergency department. A factor analytic study. *Chest.* 1993;104:1325-8.

18. Lemarchand P, Labrune S, Herer B, Huchon GJ. Cardiorespiratory arrest following peak expiratory flow measurement during attack of asthma. *Chest.* 1991;100:1168-9.

19. Hollander C, Sitkauskiene B, Sakalauskas R, Westin U, Janciauskiene SM. Serum and bronchial lavage fluid concentrations of IL-8, SLPI, sCD14 and sICAM-1 in patients with COPD and asthma. *Respir Med.* 2007;101:1947-53.

20. Higashimoto Y, Yamagata Y, Taya S, Iwata T, Okada M, Ishiguchi T, et al. Systemic inflammation in chronic obstructive pulmonary disease and asthma: similarities and differences. *Respirology.* 2008;13:128-33.

21. Snell N, Newbold P. The clinical utility of biomarkers in asthma and COPD. *Curr Opin Pharmacol.* 2008;8:222-35.

22. Leung JM, Sin DD. Biomarkers in airway diseases. *Can Respir J.* 2013;20:180-2.

23. Louhelainen N, Myllärniemi M, Rahman I, Kinnula VL. Airway biomarkers of the oxidant burden in asthma and chronic obstructive pulmonary disease: current and future perspectives. *Int J Chron Obstruct Pulmon Dis.* 2008;3:585-603.

24. Williams SG, Schmidt DK, Redd SC, Storms W; National Asthma Education and Prevention Program. Key clinical activities for quality asthma care. Recommendations of the National Asthma Education and Prevention Program. *MMWR Recomm Rep.* 2003;52:1-8.

25. Global Initiative for Asthma. Global strategy for asthma management and prevention, 2015. [online] Available from: www.ginasthma.org. [Accessed July, 2015].

26. Wilson R, Tillotson G, Ball P. Clinical studies in chronic bronchitis: a need for better definition and classification of severity. *J Antimicrob Chemother.* 1996;37:205-8.

27. Dutta EJ, Li JT. β-agonists. *Med Clin North Am.* 2002;86:991-1008.

28. O'Driscoll BR, Taylor RJ, Horsley MG, Chambers DK, Bernstein A. Nebulised salbutamol with and without ipratropium bromide in acute airflow obstruction. *Lancet.* 1989;1:1418-20.

29. Rebuck AS, Chapman KR, Abboud R, Pare PD, Kreisman H, Wolkove N, et al. Nebulized anticholinergic and sympathomimetic treatment of asthma and chronic obstructive airways disease in the emergency room. *Am J Med.* 1987;82:59-64.

30. Rodrigo GJ, Rodrigo C. First-line therapy for adult patients with acute asthma receiving a multiple-dose protocol of ipratropium bromide plus albuterol in the emergency department. *Am J Respir Crit Care Med.* 2000;161:1862-8.

31. Denniston AK, O'Brien C, Stableforth D. The use of oxygen in acute exacerbations of chronic obstructive pulmonary disease: a prospective audit of pre-hospital and hospital emergency management. *Clin Med.* 2002;2:449-51.

32. Skobeloff EM, Spivey WH, McNamara RM, Greenspon L. Intravenous magnesium sulfate for the treatment of acute asthma in the emergency department. *JAMA.* 1989;262:1210-3.

33. Tobias JD. Inhalational anesthesia: basic pharmacology, end organ effects, and applications in the treatment of status asthmaticus. *J Intensive Care Med.* 2009;24:361-71.

34. Kass JE, Terregino CA. The effect of heliox in acute severe asthma: a randomized controlled trial. *Chest.* 1999;116:296-300.

35. Hogman M, Frostell CG, Hedenstrom H, Hedenstierna G. Inhalation of nitric oxide modulates adult human bronchial tone. *Am Rev Respir Dis.* 1993;148:1474-8.

36. Burns KE, Sinuff T, Adhikari NK, Meade MO, Heels-Ansdell D, Martin CM, et al. Bilevel noninvasive positive pressure ventilation for acute respiratory failure: survey of Ontario practice. *Crit Care Med.* 2005;33:1477-83.

.37. Majid A, Hill NS. Noninvasive ventilation for acute respiratory failure. *Curr Opin Crit Care.* 2005;11:77-81.

38. British Thoracic Society Standards of Care Committee. Non-invasive ventilation in acute respiratory failure. *Thorax.* 2002;57:192-211.

39. Organized jointly by the American Thoracic Society, the European Respiratory Society, the European Society of Intensive Care Medicine, and the Société de Réanimation de Langue Française, and approved by ATS Board of Directors, December 2000. International consensus conferences in intensive care medicine. noninvasive positive pressure ventilation in acute respiratory failure. *Am J Respir Crit Care Med.* 2001;163:283-91.

40. Bott J, Carroll MP, Conway JH, Keilty SE, Ward EM, Brown AM, et al. Randomised controlled trial of nasal ventilation in acute ventilatory failure due to chronic obstructive airways disease. *Lancet.* 1993;341:1555-7.

41. Brochard L, Mancebo J, Wysocki M, Lofaso F, Conti G, Rauss A, et al. Noninvasive ventilation for acute exacerbations of chronic obstructive pulmonary disease. *N Engl J Med.* 1995;333:817-22.

42. Kramer N, Meyer TJ, Meharg J, Cece RD, Hill NS. Randomized prospective trial of noninvasive positive pressure ventilation in acute respiratory failure. *Am J Respir Crit Care Med.* 1995;151:1799-806.

43. Khilnani GC, Saikia N, Sharma SK, Pande JN, Malhotra OP. Efficacy of noninvasive positive pressure ventilation for management of COPD with acute or acute on chronic respiratory failure: a randomized controlled trial. *Am J Respir Crit Care Med.* 2002;165:A387.

44. Avdeev SN, Tret'iakov AV, Grigor'iants RA, Kutsenko MA, Chuchalin AG. Study of the use of noninvasive ventilation of the lungs in acute respiratory insufficiency due to exacerbation of chronic obstructive pulmonary disease. *Anesteziol Reanimatol.* 1998;(3):45-51.

45. Sidhu US, Behera D. Non-invasive ventilation in COPD. *Indian J Chest Dis Allied Sci.* 2000;42:105-14.

46. Plant PK, Owen JL, Elliott MW. Early use of non-invasive ventilation for acute exacerbations of chronic obstructive pulmonary disease on general respiratory wards: a multicenter randomized controlled trial. *Lancet.* 2000;355:1931-5.

47. Celikel T, Sungur M, Ceyhan B, Karakurt S. Comparison of noninvasive positive pressure ventilation with standard medical therapy in hypercapnic acute respiratory failure. *Chest.* 1998;114:1636-42.

48. Conti G, Antonelli M, Navalesi P, Rocco M, Bufi M, Spadetta G, et al. Noninvasive vs. conventional mechanical ventilation in patients with chronic obstructive pulmonary disease after failure of medical treatment in the ward: a randomized trial. *Intensive Care Med.* 2002;28:1701-7.

49. Squadrone E, Frigerio P, Fogliati C, Gregoretti C, Conti G, Antonelli M, et al. Noninvasive versus invasive ventilation in COPD patients with severe acute respiratory failure deemed to require ventilatory assistance. *Intensive Care Med.* 2004;30:1303-10.

50. Diaz GG, Alcaraz AC, Talavera JC, Pérez PJ, Rodriguez AE, Cordoba FG, et al. Noninvasive positive-pressure ventilation to treat hypercapnic coma secondary to respiratory failure. *Chest.* 2005;127:952-60.

51. Ram FS, Picot J, Lightowler J, Wedzicha JA. Non-invasive positive pressure ventilation for treatment of respiratory failure due to exacerbations of chronic obstructive pulmonary disease. *Cochrane Database Syst Rev.* 2004;(3):CD004104.

52. Rabe KF, Hurd S, Anzueto A, Barnes PJ, Buist SA, Calverley P, et al. Global strategy for the diagnosis, management, and prevention of chronic obstructive pulmonary disease: GOLD executive summary. *Am J Respir Crit Care Med.* 2007;176:532-55.

53. Meduri GU, Cook TR, Turner RE, Cohen M, Leeper KV. Noninvasive positive pressure ventilation in status asthmaticus. *Chest.* 1996;110:767-74.

54. Fernández MM, Villagra A, Blanch L, Fernández R. Non-invasive mechanical ventilation in status asthmaticus. *Intensive Care Med.* 2001;27:486-92.

55. Soroksky A, Stav D, Shpirer I. A pilot prospective, randomized, placebo-controlled trial of bilevel positive airway pressure in acute asthmatic attack. *Chest.* 2003;123(4):1018-25.

56. Holley MT, Morrissey TK, Seaberg DC, Afessa B, Wears RL. Ethical dilemmas in a randomized trial of asthma treatment: can Bayesian statistical analysis explain the results? *Acad Emerg Med.* 2001;8:1128-35.

57. Ram FS, Wellington S, Rowe B, Wedzicha JA. Non-invasive positive pressure ventilation for treatment of respiratory failure due to severe acute exacerbations of asthma. *Cochrane Database Syst Rev.* 2005;(3):CD004360.

58. Chawla R, Khilnani GC, Suri JC, Ramakrishnan N, Mani RK, Prayag S, et al. Guidelines for noninvasive ventilation in acute respiratory failure. *Indian J Crit Care Med.* 2006;10:117-47.

59. Mehta S, Hill NS. Noninvasive ventilation. *Am J Respir Crit Care Med.* 2001;163:540-77.

60. Brochard L, Mancebo J, Elliot MW. Noninvasive ventilation for acute respiratory failure. 2002;19:712-21.

61. Corbridge TC, Hall JB. The assessment and management of adults with status asthmaticus. *Am J Respir Crit Care Med.* 1995;151:1296-316.

62. Levy BD, Kitch B, Fanta CH. Medical and ventilatory management of status asthmaticus. *Intensive Care Med.* 1998;24:105-17.

63. Sarma VJ. Use of ketamine in acute severe asthma. *Acta Anaesthesiol Scand.* 1992;36:106-7.

64. Finfer SR, Garrard CS. Ventilatory support in asthma. *Br J Hosp Med.* 1993;49:357-60.

65. Georgopoulos D, Kondili E, Prinianakis G. How to set the ventilator in asthma. *Monaldi Arch Chest Dis.* 2000;55:74-83.

66. Brenner B, Corbridge T, Kazzi A. Intubation and mechanical ventilation of the asthmatic patient in respiratory failure. *Proc Am Thorac Soc.* 2009;6:371-9.

67. Brenner B, Corbridge T, Kazzi A. Intubation and mechanical ventilation of the asthmatic patient in respiratory failure. *J Allergy Clin Immunol.* 2009;124:S19-28.

68. Wildman MJ, Harrison DA, Brady AR, Rowen K. Case mix and outcomes for admissions to UK adult, general critical care units with chronic obstructive pulmonary disease: a secondary analysis of the ICNARC Case Mix Programme Database. *Crit Care.* 2005;9:S38-48.

69. Harrison DA, Brady AR, Rowen K. Case mix, outcome and length of stay for admissions to adult, general critical care units in England, Wales and Northern Ireland: the Intensive Care National Audit and Research Centre Case Mix Programme Database. *Crit Care.* 2004;8:R99-111.

70. McGhan R, Radcliff T, Fish R, Sutherland ER, Welsh C, Make B. Predictors of rehospitalization and death after a severe exacerbation of COPD. *Chest.* 2007;132:1748-55.

71. McFadden ER Jr. Acute severe asthma. *Am J Respir Crit Care Med.* 2003;168:740-59.

72. Alex CG, Tobin MJ. Ventilation of asthmatic patients. In: Barnes PJ, Grunstein MM, Leff AR, Woolcock AJ (Eds). Asthma. Philadelphia: Lippincott-Raven; 1997. pp. 1977-2003.

73. Shapiro JM. Intensive care management of status asthmaticus. *Chest.* 2001;120:1439-41.

74. Williams MH Jr. Life-threatening asthma. *Arch Int Med.* 1980;140:1604-5.

75. Wildman MJ, Sanderson C, Groves J, Reeves BC, Ayres J, Harrison D, et al. Predicting mortality for patients with exacerbations of COPD and asthma in the COPD and Asthma Outcome Study (CAOS). *QJM.* 2009;102:389-99.

76. Wildman MJ, Harrison DA, Welch CA, Sanderson C. A new measure of acute physiological derangement for patients with exacerbations of obstructive airways disease: the COPD and Asthma Physiology Score. *Respir Med.* 2007;101:1994-2002.

77. Messer B, Griffiths J, Baudouin SV. The prognostic variables predictive of mortality in patients with an exacerbation of COPD admitted to the ICU: an integrative review. *QJM.* 2012;105:115-26.

78. NHS. NICE CG101. [online] Available from: http://www.nice.org.uk/nicemedia/live/13029/49425/49425. pdf. [Accessed July, 2015].

World Clin Pulm Crit Care Med. 2016;4(1):66-79.

# Acute Respiratory Distress Syndrome

*Deepak Talwar MD DM, Arjun Khanna MD DM

Department of Pulmonary and Critical Care Medicine, Metro Center for Respiratory Diseases,
Metro Hospital and Heart Institute, Noida, Uttar Pradesh, India

## ABSTRACT

Acute respiratory distress syndrome (ARDS) is characterized by permeability pulmonary edema and refractory hypoxemia. The new Berlin definition tries to define this condition better, and to remove discrepancies associated with the older definition. The etiology of this syndrome is varied, but sepsis continues to be a major cause of ARDS and is uniformly associated with poor outcomes. Multiple pharmacological and nonpharmacological therapies have been tried in the management of ARDS, but most of these have not stood the test of time. Lung protective ventilation is still the key of better outcome in ARDS. High frequency ventilation and extracorporeal membrane oxygenation are still under debate as to their usefulness in ARDS.

## INTRODUCTION

Acute respiratory distress syndrome (ARDS) is a potentially fatal condition which manifests as rapidly progressive dyspnea, tachypnea, and hypoxemia. Usual diagnostic criteria include acute onset, and hypoxemia, bilateral pulmonary infiltrates usually in the absence of left atrial hypertension. Acute respiratory distress syndrome is usually secondary to pulmonary or extrapulmonary insults which cause massive release of inflammatory mediators, promoting neutrophil accumulation in the microcirculation of the lung. The inflammatory cells and cytokines damage the vascular endothelium and alveolar epithelium, leading to pulmonary edema, hyaline membrane formation, reduced lung compliance, and poor air exchange along the alveolar membrane. Despite multiple ventilator and pharmacological therapies, the mortality and morbidity associated with

---

*Corresponding author
*Email:* dtlung@hotmail.com

ARDS remains high. Treatment of acute respiratory distress syndrome is usually supportive and includes appropriate lung protective mechanical ventilation, prophylaxis for stress ulcers and venous thromboembolism, nutritional support, and treatment of the underlying injury. Except low tidal volume ventilation, none of the management strategies for ARDS have really stood the test of time. Elucidating the exact molecular basis of the cytokine mediated damage and the lung injury which ensues subsequently, may help us understand and manage this condition better.

## DEFINITION AND THE CONTROVERSIES

Acute respiratory distress syndrome is a clinico-radiological syndrome known since World War I as a consequence of battle trauma and now being recognized with multiple risk factors and etiologies that trigger the acute onset of respiratory insufficiency, and is associated with high morbidity and mortality. The pulmonary pathology is characterized by diffuse epithelial and endothelial cell damage, and acute exudative infiltration in the early phase, followed by variable degree of organization, fibrosis, and damage in the later phases. The exact definition of this entity has been a matter of intense debate, and different workers and centers until recently have used the American-European Consensus Conference (AECC) definition, published in 1994.[1] In this system, ARDS was defined as the acute onset of respiratory insufficiency, bilateral infiltrates on a chest radiograph, hypoxemia as defined by an arterial partial pressure of oxygen/fraction of inspired oxygen ($PaO_2/FiO_2$) ratio less than or equal to 200 mmHg, and no evidence of left atrial hypertension or a pulmonary capillary pressure less than 18 mmHg (if measured) to rule out cardiogenic pulmonary edema. The term acute lung injury (ALI) was introduced to characterize the less severe form of acute respiratory failure, and included patients with a similar clinicoradiological picture, but with $PaO_2/FiO_2$ less than or equal to 300 mmHg and greater than 200 mmHg.

This diagnostic value of this definition of ARDS has always been a matter of controversy. The different components of the definition had significant interobserver variability and thus individual workers would use the definition as per their norms, convenience, and belief. The interpretation of the chest radiographic criteria of ARDS has been reported to be poor, with high interobserver variability.[2] The oxygenation criteria, likewise, can be markedly affected by the ventilatory parameters including $FiO_2$, positive end-expiratory pressure (PEEP), and the set tidal volumes (VTs). The parameter most difficult to interpret and standardize has been the cardiac wedge pressure.

Realizing these problems, the European Society of Intensive Care Medicine along with the Society of Critical Care Medicine and the American Thoracic Society convened combined meeting of its experts in 2011 in Berlin, and formulated the Berlin definition of ARDS.[3] The key differences in this definition include:

- Removal of the term ALI to lessen confusion with one terminology rather than two as both differed in severity only
- Addition of time of onset of acute pulmonary insufficiency from the exposure to a known risk factor for ARDS to the development of the respiratory symptoms should be within 1 week in order to exclude other diseases with similar presentation but more subacute in onset
- Refined oxygenation status criteria by adding continuous positive airway pressure (CPAP) or PEEP of at least 5 cm $H_2O$ to calculate the $PaO_2/FiO_2$ ratio as patients are on some form of assisted ventilation with positive airway pressure
- Chest X-ray finding is characterized by bilateral pulmonary opacities involving at least 3 quadrants that are not fully explained by pleural effusions, atelectasis, and nodules
- Cardiogenic origin of pulmonary edema is to be excluded by objective evaluation of cardiac function with echocardiography if no identifiable known risk factors for ARDS are seen. Also, the wedge pressure measurement was abandoned because ARDS may coexist with hydrostatic edema caused by fluid overload or cardiac failure and thereby making definition more practical and easy to be applied bedside.

## EPIDEMIOLOGY

The reported incidence of ARDS is variable as expected from the case mix of different centers reporting it. Most of the available data is as per the older AECC definition and is therefore prone to inherent biases. Data from prospective US cohort studies using the AECC definition vary from 64.24 to 78.95 cases/100,000 person-years and similar figures from Northern Europe (17 cases/100,000), Spain (7.2 cases/100,000), and Australia/New Zealand (34 cases/100,000).[4-6] Large variations in ARDS incidence may be attributable to major differences in the local disease patterns and health care delivery systems. Causes of ARDS unique to the tropical regions, especially India, include malaria, leptospirosis, scrub typhus, tuberculosis, enteric fever, heat stroke, etc.[7,8] Every year, newer viral infections such as H1N1 swine flu, avian influenza, Middle East respiratory syndrome, Crimean-Congo hemorrhagic fever, etc. are added to the repertoire of organisms associated with ARDS. Mortality associated with ARDS continues to be high and death usually results from multisystem organ failure rather than respiratory failure alone. ARDS case fatality ranges from 25 to 40%, which appears to have improved over 50–70% reported earlier.[9]

## ETIOPATHOGENESIS

The identifiable risk factors for the development of ARDS can be grouped as insults ensuing from either direct or indirect injury to the lung (Table 1). Sepsis is probably the single most commonly identified cause of ARDS encountered in intensive care, and is usually associated with poor outcome. Whatever being the cause of ARDS, trauma, aspiration, sepsis, or any primary cause it leads to injury to the alveolar epithelium and capillary endothelium which leads to a leakage of protein-rich plasma into alveoli.[10] These plasma proteins then activate procoagulant and proinflammatory pathways leading to formation of fibrinous and purulent exudates. Proinflammatory cytokines cause intense inflammation, which leads to cell pneumocyte injury and death. Many of these cytokines promote fibrogenesis leading to development of permanent fibrosis and chronic respiratory failure.

Accumulation of extravascular lung water in the acute phase is the basis of physiological derangements of ARDS manifesting as hypoxemia with lower respiratory compliance and as the exudative fluid floods more alveoli, severe shunt develops leading to development of refractory hypoxemia.[11] Many of remaining normal alveoli collapse from increase in surface tension worsening further oxygenation.

Increased pulmonary vascular resistance is commonly seen in patients with ARDS secondary to hypoxia-induced reduction in the luminal diameter of the vascular bed, and thrombotic occlusion of the microvasculature.[12] The decrease in respiratory compliance is particularly more severe in direct forms of ARDS such as pneumonia. The increase in alveolar surface tension is being considered to develop from the increased surface forces generated by a decrease in surfactant activity. Further, unaffected healthy lungs may get over distended and can lead to volutrauma seen in ventilator-induced lung injury.

Hence, phases of ARDS can be further subdivided into exudative, proliferative, and fibrotic phases, though they may not occur sequentially.[10] The exudative phase typically occupies the first week and is characterized by intense inflammation and widespread pulmonary damage. The proliferative phase starts from second week

| Table 1: Risk Factors for the Development of Acute Respiratory Distress Syndrome | |
| --- | --- |
| **Direct causes** | **Indirect causes** |
| • Pneumonia | • Sepsis, secondary to multiple infections |
| • Aspiration of gastric contents | • Acute pancreatitis |
| • Trauma and lung contusion | • Blood transfusion reactions |
| • Drowning | • Drug overdose |
| • Toxic inhalations | • Burns |
| • Lung surgery | • Polytrauma |
| | • Cardiopulmonary bypass |

to fourth week and characterized by organization of the intra-alveolar exudates with proliferation of type II alveolar cells, fibroblasts, and myofibroblasts. The fibrotic phase is seen in patients who survive past 3 or 4 weeks. On pathological examination, alveolar septa are expanded and airspaces filled with sparsely cellular connective tissue, and remodeling can progress to the point of complete airspace obliteration and fibrosis leading to chronic respiratory failure.

## MANAGEMENT

Numerous trials have been conducted in patients with ARDS, but great advances in the care of the patients are still lacking and supportive therapies remain the mainstay in the management of ARDS. Various pharmacological and ventilatory strategies have been tried in the management of ARDS (Table 2). However, most of these have not stood the test of time and most have shown little or no mortality benefit.

Perhaps, the most important key in the management of ARDS lies in the prevention of further lung injury, this includes injury caused by invasive mechanical ventilation. In accordance with the same, lung protective ventilation deserves special mention (Figures 1 and 2).

### Lung Protective Ventilation Strategies

Substantial data now exists demonstrating that mechanical ventilation, especially in the setting of lung injury, can worsen the lung injury and add to systemic inflammation. The ARDS lung is a heterogeneous lung. On one hand there are alveoli, full of inflammatory exudates, which are tough to ventilate and on the other hand there are the normal alveoli, which may get damaged when high pressure/volume strategies to ventilate the lung are used. The key to ventilating an ARDS lung lies in protective mechanical ventilation, which aims at preventing the downward spiral of further lung injury. This is easier said then done. Very often, the poorly compliant lungs of ARDS patients are extremely difficult to ventilate, and mortality remains high, even in the best of centers. The most important evidence supporting lung protective ventilation comes from the National Institutes of Health (NIH)-sponsored multicenter study of patients with ARDS.[13] In this landmark trial, patients randomized to receive a lower VT [4–6 mL/kg predict body weight (PBW), and maintenance of plateau pressure (Pplat) between 25 and 30 cm $H_2O$] had a survival benefit. Mortality was reduced by 40% in the conventional arm to 31% in the low VT arm (CI, 2.4–15.3% difference between groups). The group ventilated with lung protective strategies demonstrated lower circulating cytokines, such as interleukin-6 (IL-6) levels demonstrating lesser systemic spillover of the pulmonary inflammation, which attributed to multiple organ dysfunction syndrome (MODS) and mortality in ARDS (Figures 3 and 4).

**Table 2: Summary of Various Therapies Tested and Recommended in Acute Respiratory Distress Syndrome**

| Intervention | End Points | Highest level of evidence | Recommendation |
|---|---|---|---|
| Surfactant: pooled data | Mortality Ventilator-free days | I | No |
| Surfactant: protein-free surfactants | Mortality Ventilator-free days | I | No |
| Surfactant: protein-contaning surfactants | Mortality Ventilator-free days | I | No |
| Nitric oxide | Mortality Oxygenation | I | No Yes |
| Inhaled prostacyclins | Oxygenation | V | Yes |
| Vasodilators: IV PGE 1 | Mortality Ventilator-free days | II | No |
| Vasodilators: liposomal IV PGE | Mortality Ventilator-free days | I | No |
| High-dose methylprednisolone for prevention of ARDS in patients at risk | Incidence of ARDS | I | No |
| High-dose methylprednisolone for early therapy of ARDS | Mortality Severity of lung injury | II | No |
| High-dose methylprednisolone for subacute (late) phase of ARDS | Mortality Ventilator-free days | I | No |
| Ketoconazole | Mortality Ventilator-free days | I | No |
| Lisofylline | Mortality Ventilator-free days | I | No |
| Pentoxifylline | Safety | V | No |
| N-acetylcysteine | Mortality Ventilator-free days | II | No |
| Procysteine | Mortality Ventilator-free days | II | No |

IV PGE, intravenous infusion of prostaglandin E; ARDS, acute respiratory distress syndrome.

At the end of each respiratory cycle, the alveoli collapse. The next inspiratory effort, therefore, has to be strong enough to open all the alveoli. This would entail application of higher pressures to open up the heterogeneous ARDS lung and cause more injury. Thus, came the concept of PEEP. The concept of PEEP is both fascinating and controversial. While the exact level and utility of PEEP required to ventilate a patient of ARDS remains controversial, several trials try and unlock

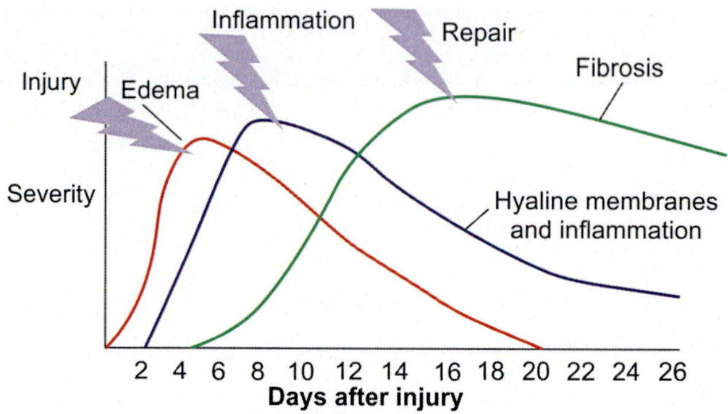



**Figure 1:** Window of opportunity to intervene with targeting edema in first phase, anti-inflammatory therapies in second phase and antifibrotic strategies in third phase.

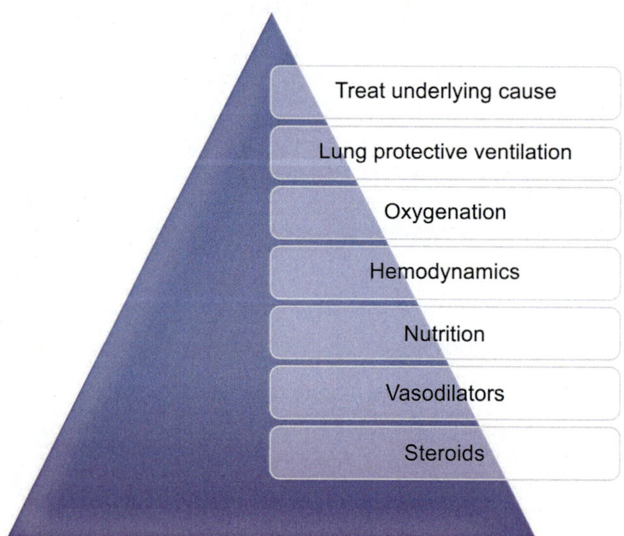



**Figure 2:** Many facets of management of acute respiratory distress syndrome, but only few are without controversies.

this mystery. The most often quoted studies by Amato et al.[14] and Villar et al.[15] examined the effect of a strategy that minimized VT, adopted lung recruitment maneuvers, and applied a level of PEEP above the closing pressure of the lung and the intervention arms decreased mortality, but the studies were criticized due to relatively small sample sizes and relatively high mortality in the control arms. The ARDS Network (ARDSNet) performed a second large clinical trial comparing lower versus higher levels of PEEP (ALVEOLI study)[14] but the trial was stopped early for futility, showing a trend for worse outcome in the higher PEEP arm,

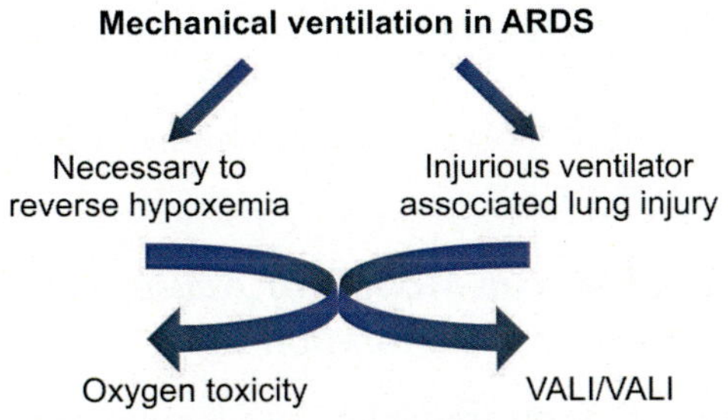



ARDS, acute respiratory distress syndrome; VALI ventilation-associated lung injury.

**Figure 3:** Ventilation in ARDS is double-edged sword which needs to ventilate to archive adequate oxygenation but simultaneously needs to do it so as to minimize toxicity as well as ventilator-associated injury.

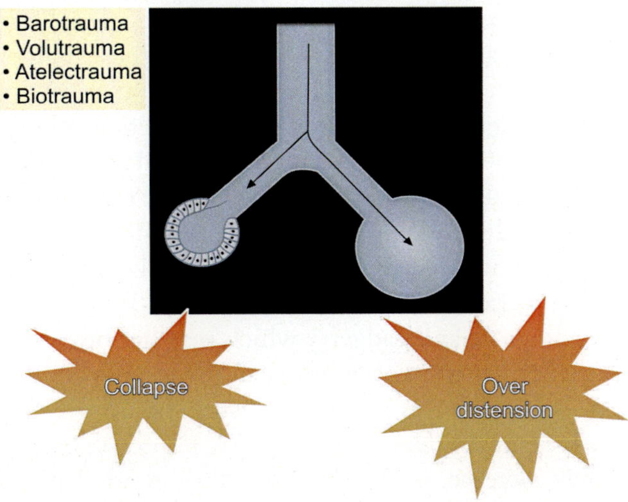



**Figure 4:** Types of ventilation-associated lung injury which may be due to pressure, volume, stretch, or inflammatory mediators induced.

although there was an imbalance in patient characteristics at baseline favoring the control arm; the mean age of the higher PEEP arm was higher ($54 \pm 17$ vs. $49 \pm 17$, $p < 0.05$), the mean $PaO_2/FiO_2$ was lower ($151 \pm 67$ vs. $165 \pm 77$, $p < 0.05$), and there was a trend toward higher Acute Physiology and Chronic Health Evaluation III scores, at baseline. The French EXPRESS study addressed the superiority of an open lung approach in which PEEP was titrated to the highest value possible keeping Pplat less than 28–30 cm $H_2O$ with control arm PEEP set between 5 and 9 cm $H_2O$ and VT was less than 6 mL/kg PBW in both groups.[16] Patient treated according to the open lung approach had significantly more ventilator-free days and organ-failure free days; however, in hospital 28-day and 60-day mortality were not different between the study groups. But it is worth mentioning that patients who now would be considered to have moderate-to-severe lung injury (P/F <200) tended to have lower 28-day mortality in the higher PEEP group compared to patients treated with lower PEEP.

### Other Nonconventional Rescue Modes for Acute Respiratory Distress Syndrome Ventilation

Prone position ventilation, high frequency oscillatory ventilation (HFOV), and extracorporeal membrane oxygenation (ECMO) are the three most quoted and talked about methods for patients with refractory ARDS, where the conventional therapies have failed. We do not know weather these strategies actually work as literature is replete with contradictory reports. Our personal experience is that while these strategies do improve oxygenation transiently, the mortality benefit is not apparent. Also, most of these interventions require special units which have sufficient experience in managing patients, who are on these high end therapeutic modalities.

The prone positioning exploits effect of gravity and repositioning of the heart in the thorax to recruit the lung bases to improve ventilation perfusion matching thereby improving arterial oxygenation. Workers have demonstrated that prone ventilation was associated with a decrease in (37.8 vs. 46.1%) 28-day mortality in the subgroup of patients with severe hypoxemia, but given the small numbers in the subgroup, a definitive conclusion cannot be drawn.[17] Prone position ventilation requires special nursing care and gadgetry which may not be easily available.

High frequency oscillatory ventilation is an extreme form of lung protective ventilation, where the patient is ventilated using volumes equivalent to dead space ventilation. Despite evidence that HFOV improves oxygenation, it does not reduce, and may increase, in-hospital mortality in adult patients with adult respiratory distress syndrome compared with a ventilation strategy of low VT and high PEEP. A number of studies and meta-analyses have examined whether HFOV reduces mortality. In the largest, multicenter trial, the Oscillation for Acute Respiratory Distress Syndrome Treated Early (OSCILLATE) investigators randomly assigned adult patients with new-onset moderate-to-severe ARDS to HFOV or to an ARDSNet ventilation strategy.[18] This well-designed study was terminated early after enrollment of 548 of a planned 1,200 patients. The study was terminated for harm with an in-hospital mortality of 47% in the HFOV arm and 35% in the ARDSNet arm (relative risk of death with HFOV, 1.33; 95% CI 1.09–1.64; p = 0.005). Thus, HFOV cannot be recommended as the initial treatment strategy for adult patients with ARDS.

The OSCAR trial, involving nearly 800 patients in the UK, also failed to demonstrate a mortality benefit at 30 days although the detrimental effect of HFOV on mortality observed in the OSCILLATE trial above was not in evidence.[19]

In patients with severe ARDS where conventional methods have failed, ECMO has been considered as possible rescue therapy. ECMO provides lung rest, while the primary injury abates and the ventilatory work is taken care of by the ECMO apparatus. The utility of ECMO in ARDS was best demonstrated during the H1N1 pandemics, where world over traditional strategies aimed at ventilating ARDS patients were associated with dismal results. Despite earlier negative trials, the Conventional Care versus Extracorporeal Support in Adult Respiratory Failure (CESAR) study showed benefit of extracorporeal life support in severe ARDS.[20] This randomized controlled trial (RCT) had 180 patients randomized to venovenous ECMO (after transfer to a specialized center) or conventional mechanical ventilation (in regional centers). The former group had a better 6 months survival than the latter one, but it is a possibility that the ECMO patients received a best practice treatment in specialized centers versus control group which was treated as per the discretion of physicians at multiple nonspecialized hospitals.

## Pharmacological and Other Supportive Therapy of Acute Respiratory Distress Syndrome

Another controversy in the management of these patients is the exact fluid therapy to be used in them. A fluid restrictive strategy was evaluated by ARDSNet-sponsored RCT aimed to limit the net fluid balance in ARDS patients without shock and renal failure requiring replacement therapy. Mortality at 60 days was not different between the two study groups. However, patients randomized to fluid restriction had more mechanical ventilation-free days and a lower intensive care unit (ICU) length of stay compared to those patients randomized to liberal fluid intake. The two study groups were different in terms of cumulative fluid balance; in particular, the liberal fluid group had positive fluid balance of 7 L in at 1 week with 1 L of net fluid gain each day.[21]

In patients with severe ARDS ($PaO_2/FiO_2$ <150), 48 hours administration of nondepolarizing neuromuscular blocking agent (NMBA) cisatracurium has been shown to improve oxygenation, and adjusted 90-day survival, as well as decreasing duration of mechanical ventilation and barotrauma, without increasing muscle weakness.[22] These agents also decrease levels of both pulmonary and systemic proinflammatory mediators. However, in view of the potential side effects of critical illness neuromyopathy, use of NMBAs should be limited to severely hypoxemic patients for a brief period only (Figure 5).

Inhaled nitric oxide for its pulmonary vasodilator effects has been suggested to treat refractory hypoxemia by improving ventilation-perfusion matching. Meta-analyses indicate that inhaled nitric oxide improves oxygenation over a 24-hour period of treatment. However, again no mortality benefit was demonstrated.[23]

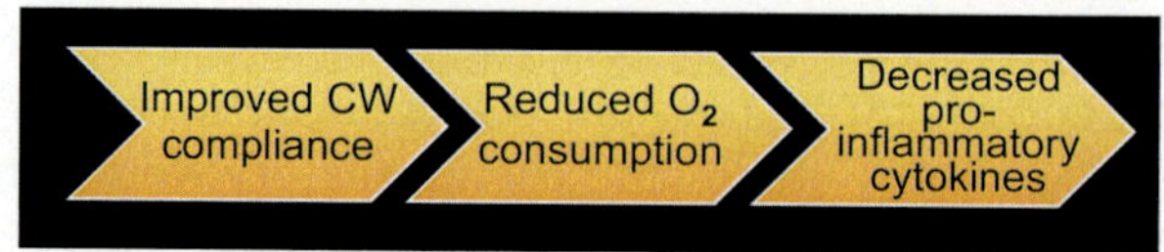



**Figure 5:** Neuromuscular blockade (NMB) is used in 25–55% of patients with acute respiratory distress syndrome and has more than one effect with potential to improve oxygenation which is seen by single dose of NMB.

But the incidence of MODS increased with the use of nitric oxide. This problem with the use of nitric oxide is, similar to other agents tried in ARDS, where the oxygenation improved transiently, but the mortality did not change.

Probably no other agent has evoked more controversy in the management of ARDS than glucocorticosteroids. The literature is replete with contrasting studies which promote or discourage the use of steroids and cause confusion for the practicing intensivist. Impressive trials with preventive corticosteroids, mostly using high doses of methyl prednisolone, showed negative results with patients in treatment arm, showing higher mortality and rate of ARDS development. While trials of corticosteroids in early ARDS showed variable results, somewhat, favoring use of these agents to reduce associated morbidities. In late stage of ARDS, these drugs have no benefits and are associated with adverse outcome. Use of corticosteroids in patients with early ARDS showed equivocal results in decreasing mortality; however, there is evidence that these drugs reduce organ dysfunction score, lung injury score, ventilator requirement and ICU stay. However, most of these trials are small, having a significant heterogeneity regarding study design, etiology of ARDS, and dosage of corticosteroids.[24,25] Further research involving large-scale trials on relatively homogeneous cohort is necessary to establish the role of corticosteroids for this condition.

### Additional Therapies

Various pharmacologic therapies have been investigated for the reduction of pulmonary damage in ALI/ARDS. Agents studied include ketoconazole, pentoxifylline, and N-acetylcysteine (NAC), but none of these therapies has demonstrated a reduction in mortality.[26-28] Ketoconazole, a synthetic imidazole with anti-inflammatory properties, was evaluated in a randomized, double-blind, placebo-controlled study of 234 patients with ALI/ARDS.[26] The study concluded ketoconazole did not improve lung function or reduce mortality or duration of mechanical ventilation. The vasodilator pentoxifylline was studied in a pilot trial involving six patients with severe ARDS. The trial concluded that large doses of intravenous (IV) pentoxifylline induced small hemodynamic changes without any worsening of pulmonary gas exchange. NAC has been studied based on its antioxidant properties, which provide protective effects against acute pulmonary injury. A double-blind, placebo-controlled study of 48 patients found that treatment with IV NAC (70 mg/kg) decreased the number of days of ARDS without affecting overall mortality.[28]

## CONCLUSION

Adoption of the new Berlin definition may be useful to better classify patients according to severity and prognosis. ARDS still continues to be a difficult clinical condition to treat. Most of the trials of various ventilatory and nonventilatory strategies have yielded negative results with no mortality benefit. Supportive therapies represent the mainstay of treatment of ARDS, whereas the limitation of end-inspiratory lung stretch has been clearly demonstrated to reduce the ARDS-associated mortality. The pathogenesis of this disease condition is complex and future therapy such as gene therapy and mesenchymal stem cells, targeting the molecular pathology may yield positive results by modulating the pathophysiological mechanisms.

### Editor's Comment

*Acute respiratory distress syndrome (ARDS) is an entity which has evolved in its definition, pathophysiology, and treatment and ventilator strategy over the last decade. From the traditional definition of acute lung injury and ARDS, we have now a more comprehensive and objective Berlin definition of ARDS. Our understandings of the disease and its short- and long-term effects on the lung have become clearer. The management of ARDS, especially the ventilator strategy, has evolved dramatically over the last decade. Standard protocols using the studies done by the Acute Respiratory Distress Syndrome Network group have been developed and the ventilatory management of ARDS has become more streamlined. In patients not responding and requiring high $FiO_2$, many strategies have been tried. High frequency oscillatory ventilation showed initial promise in small studies but subsequently two studies—the OSCILLATE and OSCAR trials—showed no benefit and even harm (OSCILLATE showed increased mortality with high frequency oscillatory ventilation). Extracorporeal membrane oxygenation has also emerged as a useful alternative in managing refractory hypoxemia in ARDS. A lot of data after the H1N1 pandemic showed this modality to be useful and has started picking up in India as well. Controversy about the use of steroids in early and late phase of ARDS still persists. Major changes in the way we manage ARDS over the last decade has led to a significant improvement in survival in these patients.*

***Randeep Guleria***

## REFERENCES


1. Bernard GR, Artigas A, Brigham KL, Carlet J, Falke K, Hudson L, et al. The American-European Consensus Conference on ARDS. Definitions, mechanisms, relevant outcomes, and clinical trial coordination. *Am J Respir Crit Care Med.* 1994;149:818-24.
2. Meade MO, Cook RJ, Guyatt GH, Groll R, Kachura JR, Bedard M, et al. Interobserver variation in interpreting chest radiographs for the diagnosis of acute respiratory distress syndrome. *Am J Respir Crit Care Med.* 2000;161:85-90.
3. ARDS Definition Task Force, Ranieri VM, Rubenfeld GD, Thompson BT, Ferguson ND, Caldwell E, et al. Acute respiratory distress syndrome: the Berlin Definition. *JAMA.* 2012;307:2526-33.
4. Luhr OR, Antonsen K, Karlsson M, Aardal S, Thorsteinsson A, Frostell CG, et al. Incidence and mortality after acute respiratory failure and acute respiratory distress syndrome in Sweden, Denmark, and Iceland. The ARF study group. *Am J Respir Crit Care Med.* 1999;159:1849-61.
5. Villar J, Blanco J, Anon JM, Santos-Bouza A, Blanch L, Ambros A, et al. The ALIEN study: incidence and outcome of acute respiratory distress syndrome in the era of lung protective ventilation. *Intensive Care Med.* 2011;37:1932-41.
6. Bersten AD, Edibam C, Hunt T, Moran J; Australian and New Zealand Intensive Care Society Clinical Trials Group. Incidence and mortality of acute lung injury and the acute respiratory distress syndrome in three Australian states. *Am J Respir Crit Care Med.* 2002;165:443-8.
7. Mohan A, Sharma SK, Bollineni S. Acute lung injury and acute respiratory distress syndrome in malaria. *J Vector Borne Dis.* 2008;45:179-93.
8. Limaye CS, Londhey VA, Nabar ST. The study of complications of vivax malaria in comparison with falciparum malaria in Mumbai. *J Assoc Physicians India.* 2012;60:15-8.
9. Milberg JA, Davis DR, Steinberg KP, Hudson LD. Improved survival of patients with acute respiratory distress syndrome (ARDS): 1983–1993. *JAMA.* 1995;273:306-9.
10. Tomashefski JF Jr. Pulmonary pathology of acute respiratory distress syndrome. *Clin Chest Med.* 2000;21:435-66.
11. Piantadosi CA, Schwartz DA. The acute respiratory distress syndrome. *Ann Intern Med.* 2004;141:460-70.
12. Villar J, Blazquez MA, Lubillo S, Quintana J, Manzano JL. Pulmonary hypertension in acute respiratory failure. *Crit Care Med.* 1989;17:523-6.
13. Ventilation with lower tidal volumes as compared with traditional tidal volumes for acute lung injury and the acute respiratory distress syndrome. The Acute Respiratory Distress Syndrome Network. *N Engl J Med.* 2000;342:1301-8.
14. Amato MB, Barbas CS, Medeiros DM, Magaldi RB, Schettino GP, Lorenzi-Filho G, et al. Effect of a protective-ventilation strategy on mortality in the acute respiratory distress syndrome. *N Engl J Med.* 1998;338:347-54.
15. Villar J, Kacmarek RM, Pérez-Méndez L, Aguirre-Jaime A. A high positive end-expiratory pressure, low tidal volume ventilatory strategy improves outcome in persistent acute respiratory distress syndrome: a randomized, controlled trial. *Crit Care Med.* 2006;34:1311-8.
16. Mercat A, Richard JC, Vielle B, Jaber S, Osman D, Diehl JL, et al. Positive end-expiratory pressure setting in adults with acute lung injury and acute respiratory distress syndrome: a randomized controlled trial. *JAMA.* 2008;299:646-55.
17. Taccone P, Pesenti A, Latini R, Polli F, Vagginelli F, Mietto C, et al. Prone positioning in patients with moderate and severe acute respiratory distress syndrome: a randomized controlled trial. *JAMA.* 2009;302:1977-84.
18. Ferguson ND, Cook DJ, Guyatt GH, Mehta S, Hand L, Austin P, et al. High-frequency oscillation in early acute respiratory distress syndrome. *N Engl J Med.* 2013;368:795-805.
19. Young D, Lamb SE, Shah S, MacKenzie I, Tunnicliffe W, Lall R, et al. High-frequency oscillation for acute respiratory distress syndrome. *N Engl J Med.* 2013;368:806-13.
20. Peek GJ, Mugford M, Tiruvoipati R, Wilson A, Allen E, Thalanany MM, et al. Efficacy and economic assessment of conventional ventilatory support versus extracorporeal membrane oxygenation for severe adult respiratory failure (CESAR): a multicentre randomised controlled trial. *Lancet.* 2009;374:1351-63.

21. National Heart, Lung, and Blood Institute Acute Respiratory Distress Syndrome (ARDS) Clinical Trials Network, Wiedemann HP, Wheeler AP, Bernard GR, Thompson BT, Hayden D, et al. Comparison of two fluid-management strategies in acute lung injury. *N Engl J Med.* 2006;354:2564-75.
22. Papazian L, Forel JM, Gacouin A, Penot-Ragon C, Perrin G, Loundou A, et al. Neuromuscular blockers in early acute respiratory distress syndrome. *N Engl J Med.* 2010;363:1107-16.
23. Adhikari NK, Burns KE, Friedrich JO, Granton JT, Cook DJ, Meade MO. Effect of nitric oxide on oxygenation and mortality in acute lung injury: systematic review and meta-analysis. *BMJ.* 2007;334:779.
24. Meduri GU, Headley AS, Golden E, Carson SJ, Umberger RA, Kelso T, et al. Effect of prolonged methylprednisolone therapy in unresolving acute respiratory distress syndrome: a randomized controlled trial. *JAMA.* 1998;280:159-65.
25. Annane D, Sebille V, Bellissant E; Ger-Inf-05 Study Group. Effect of low doses of corticosteroids in septic shock patients with or without early acute respiratory distress syndrome. *Crit Care Med.* 2006;34:22-30.
26. Ketoconazole for early treatment of acute lung injury and acute respiratory distress syndrome. a randomized controlled trial. The ARDS Network. *JAMA.* 2000;283:1995-2002.
27. Montravers P, Fagon JY, Gilbert C, Blanchet F, Novara A, Chastre J. Pilot study of cardiopulmonary risk from pentoxifylline in adult respiratory distress syndrome. *Chest.* 1993;103:1017-22.
28. Bernard GR, Wheeler AP, Arons MM, Morris PE, Paz HL, Russell JA, et al. A trial of antioxidants N-acetylcysteine and procysteine in ARDS. The antioxidant in ARDS Study Group. *Chest.* 1997;112:164-72.

World Clin Pulm Crit Care Med. 2016;4(1):80-100.

# Pulmonary Thromboembolism

*Devasahayam J Christopher BSc DTCD DNB FICS FRCP FCCP,
Richa Gupta MD FCCP

Department of Pulmonary Medicine, Christian Medical College and Hospital
Vellore, Tamil Nadu, India

## ABSTRACT

Pulmonary thromboembolism commonly results form deep venous thrombosis attributable to the triad of factors related to clot formation (Virchow's triad): venous stasis, increased blood coagulability and injury to the vein wall. Evaluating the likelihood of pulmonary embolism (PE) in an individual patient according to the clinical presentation is of utmost importance not only for the interpretation of the diagnostic test results but, also for the selection of an appropriate diagnostic strategy. When PE is diagnosed, inpatient therapy with initial bed rest for 24–48 hours is often recommended.

Anticoagulation is the mainstay of treatment for acute PE. Stable PE can be managed in hospital or on an outpatient basis. Thrombolytic therapy is recommended as the first-line treatment for patients with massive PE (hemodynamic compromise/imminent cardiac arrest). Thrombolytic therapy should be instituted at the earliest in such patients provided there are no contraindications pertaining to risk of bleeding. Surgical embolectomy should be reserved for a select group of patients who have massive PE with hemodynamic instability requiring cardiopulmonary resuscitation, for those who have failed thrombolytic therapy or have contraindications to its use.

## INTRODUCTION

Venous thromboembolism encompasses pulmonary embolism (PE) and deep vein thrombosis (DVT) which are different manifestations of the same disease. Recent advances in the diagnostic strategies, pharmacotherapeutics and surgical

---

*Corresponding author
*Email:* djchris@cmcvellore.ac.in

managements have decreased mortality from venous thromboembolic disease significantly in the past few decades.[1]

## EPIDEMIOLOGY

In most cases, PE is a consequence of DVT. Among patients with proximal DVT, about 50% have an associated, usually clinically asymptomatic PE on lung scan.[2] In about 70% of patients with PE, DVT can be found in the lower limbs if sensitive diagnostic methods are used.[3,4] The risk of death related to the initial acute episode or to recurrent PE is greater in patients who present with PE than in those who present with DVT.[5] According to prospective cohort studies, the acute case fatality rate for PE ranges from 7 to 11%.[6] Also, recurrent episodes are about 3 times more likely to be PE after an initial PE than after an initial DVT (60% vs. 20%).[6] The overall age- and sex-adjusted annual incidence of venous thromboembolic disease is approximately 1–2 cases per 1,000 persons and is considered strongly age dependent and the incidence rises to about 1% per year in persons greater than 75 years of age.[7,8]

A recent epidemiological study confirmed that venous thromboembolism (VTE) is a major public health burden with an estimated 370,000 related deaths in 2004 in six European countries.[9] Moreover, PE may lead to chronic thromboembolic pulmonary hypertension, which can be severely disabling.[10-11] Pulmonary embolism has been shown by autopsy studies to be the cause of mortality in 10% of all hospital deaths and contributing to mortality in further ten percent. Two-thirds of the cases of PE are unsuspected and unconfirmed ante-mortem. Furthermore, it is well known that only one-third of the cases suspected to be PE on the basis of clinical symptoms are confirmed of the diagnosis after investigations (Figure 1).

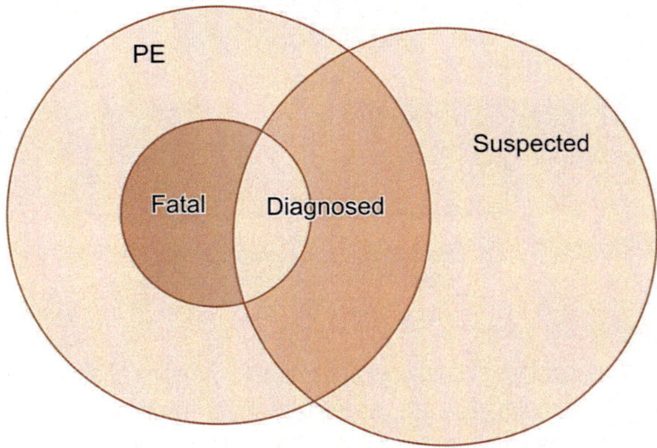


**Figure 1:** Relationship between suspected and diagnosed pulmonary embolism (PE).

## PATHOPHYSIOLOGY

The pathophysiology of PE includes formation of DVT and subsequent embolization into the pulmonary arteries. Current evidence confirms that the triad of factors related to clot formation (Virchow's triad): venous stasis, increased blood coagulability, and injury to the vein wall are the most important factors in the pathogenesis of VTE. The most common source of pulmonary emboli is thrombosis in the deep veins of the lower limbs, particularly between the knee and the inguinal ligament. PE is infrequently due to thrombosis of the pelvic veins, veins of the upper extremities or other organ systems (e.g., hepatic and renal veins). Release of vasoactive substances like serotonin from the platelets and the blockade of the pulmonary artery by the clot cause an elevation of pulmonary vascular resistance. This results in an increase in right ventricular work load, leading to a redistribution of blood flow and if the increase in right ventricular work load is excessive, it may result in right ventricular failure (Figure 2).

Airway obstruction resulting from the reflex bronchoconstriction further contributes to the ventilation-perfusion (V/Q) mismatch. After about 24 hours, there is depletion of surfactant; this may result in atelectasis and edema in the affected area.

Although the site of the clot and the extent of obstruction determine the severity of the disease and the outcome, in the presence of pre-existing cardiopulmonary disease, a small embolic event in the pulmonary artery may

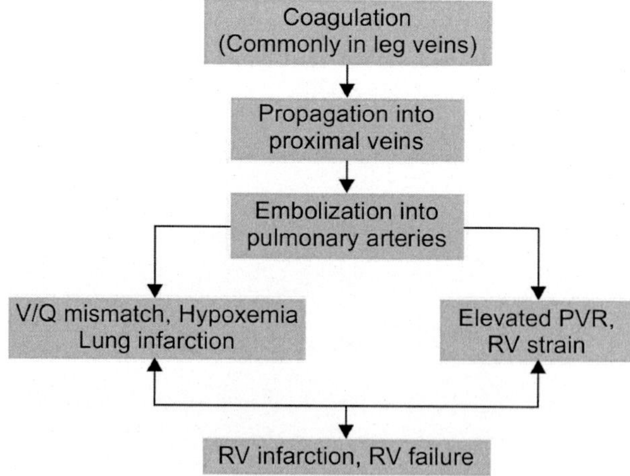


PVR, pulmonary vascular resistance; RV, right ventricular.

**Figure 2:** Pathophysiology of pulmonary embolism. Formation of deep vein thrombosis and embolization into pulmonary arteries leads to acute increase in pulmonary vascular resistance, which increases the demand on the right ventricle and may decrease the cardiac output. This combination of effects can lead to right ventricular dysfunction, infarction, and even cardiac arrest.

result in serious consequences. Conversely, a major occlusion in one of the main pulmonary arteries may have lesser consequences in a person with a normal pre-existing cardiopulmonary status.

## RISK FACTORS

Venous thromboembolism is currently considered to be the result of an interaction between patient-related and setting-related risk factors.[12] Patient-related predisposing factors are usually permanent, whereas setting-related risk factors are more often temporary (Table 1). However, the predictive values of these factors are not equal and VTE can occur in patients without any identifiable predisposing factors.

### Surgery and Fractures

Recent surgery and fractures, particularly of the femur and tibia, pose an increased risk. In surgical patients, the high-risk groups are those that have major high-risk operations performed for abdominal or pelvic malignancy and major orthopedic

| Table 1: Risk Factors for Pulmonary Embolism | | |
|---|---|---|
| | **Major risk factors** | **Minor risk factors** |
| Surgery and fractures | • Abdominal/pelvic surgery<br>• Hip/knee replacement<br>• Postoperative ICU care<br>• Bone fractures especially of tibia and femur | • Oral contraceptive pills<br>• Hormone replacement therapy<br>• Myocardial infarction<br>• Congestive cardiac failure<br>• Congenital heart disease |
| Malignancy | • Pancreatic<br>• Bronchial<br>• Genitourinary<br>• Stomach and colon<br>• Breast<br>• Advanced/metastatic | • Superficial venous thrombosis<br>• Indwelling central vein catheter<br>• Chronic obstructive airways disease<br>• Increasing age<br>• Occult malignancy<br>• Thrombotic disorders |
| Obstetrics | • Pregnancy-late<br>• Puerperium<br>• Cesarean section | • Long distance sedentary travel<br>• Obesity |
| Immobilization (especially lower limb) | • Plaster of Paris cast<br>• Paralysis<br>• Hospitalization<br>• Institutional care | |
| Others | • Previous proven VTE | |

ICU, intensive care unit; VTE, venous thromboembolism.

surgery, or any surgery requiring intensive care. The likely causative factors are immobility and liberation of clotting factors.

## Malignancy

Although the exact mechanism for this is unknown, abnormalities of hemostasis occur in patients with neoplastic disease. A well-known example of this is the association of thrombophlebitis migrans with gastrointestinal tract malignant disease. The association of VTE is seen most often with pancreatic cancer, followed in the order of frequency by carcinomas of the bronchial tree, genitourinary tract, colon, stomach, and breast.

## Pregnancy and Puerperium

Venous thromboembolism is one of the leading causes of maternal morbidity and mortality. About two-thirds of these VTE cases occur during pregnancy and one-third postpartum. A recent case-control study showed that the risk of VTE was increased fivefold [odds ratio (OR) 4.6, 95% confidence interval (CI) 2.7–7.8] during pregnancy and increased 60-fold (OR 60.1, 95% CI 26.5–135.9) during the first 3 months following delivery compared with nonpregnant women.[13] The risk was highest in the third trimester of pregnancy and during the first 6 weeks after delivery.

## Immobilization

Immobilization for more than a week is an important risk factor. Diminished muscle activity in the lower limbs reduces venous return, facilitating accumulation of activated clotting factors.

## Oral Contraceptive Therapy

Most oral contraceptive pills (OCPs) consist of a combination of estrogen and progestogen. The reduction in use of estrogen over time and this has reduced the risk of VTE in females. However, there is still a 2- to 5-fold increased risk, with the risk being highest during first year of use.[14]

## Cardiorespiratory Disorders

The source of the emboli in these diseases is also the veins of the lower limbs, rather than the heart itself. In these situations, the risk of clot formation in the leg veins is probably enhanced by the reduction in the peripheral blood flow. VTE has been reported to be over 3 times more common in patients with heart disease (aged 30 years or more) than in age matched controls.

## Inherited Causes

Deficiencies of natural coagulation inhibitors such as antithrombin, protein C and protein S are strong risk factors for VTE but these deficiencies are rare and account for only 1% of all cases of VTE. Factor V Leiden and prothrombin (factor II) G20210A are two more common genetic variants that have been consistently found to be associated with VTE, but still explain only a small proportion of VTE cases.

## Age

Age is an important risk factor. In one series, 88.5% of the patients diagnosed with PE were aged 40 years or more.

## CLINICAL FEATURES

The clinical presentation of PE can vary widely from one patient to another. Evaluating the likelihood of PE in an individual patient according to the clinical presentation is of utmost importance not only for the interpretation of the diagnostic test results but, also for the selection of an appropriate diagnostic strategy.[15]

Suspicion of PE is raised by clinical symptoms such as dyspnea, chest pain and syncope, either alone or in combination. In several series, dyspnea, tachypnea, or chest pain were present in more than 90% of patients with PE.[16,17] The initial presentation usually falls into one of the three following categories:[18]

1.  Pulmonary infarction syndrome: the patients who fall in this category present with dyspnea and pleuritic chest pain. The severity of PE in these patients is deemed to be mild.
2.  Isolated dyspnea: in these patients, the only symptom is acute shortness of breath. These patients are often hypoxic, and PE is deemed to be moderate. This presentation probably is encountered in roughly one-fifth of the patients.
3.  Circulatory collapse: patients in this category present with circulatory collapse, characterized by shock or syncope. PE is deemed to be severe.

It is good to keep the following factors in mind during clinical assessment of a patient with suspected PE:

- Pleuritic chest pain, with or without dyspnea, is one of the most frequent presentations of PE. Moderate to large embolism may be associated with retrosternal; angina-like chest pain, which may reflect right ventricular ischemia
- The onset of dyspnea may at times be insidious in onset, progressive over several weeks, and the diagnosis of PE is considered by the absence of other causes of dyspnea
- Syncope is a rare presentation of PE and may indicate a severely reduced hemodynamic reserve.

On physical examination, tachypnea is the most common sign. Other signs include tachycardia, crackles, fever, diaphoresis, cyanosis, parasternal heave, loud pulmonary component of the second heart sound, third or fourth heart sound, wheezes, pleural friction rub, hepatomegaly, and hepato-jugular reflux. But these findings are common to several cardiopulmonary disorders and so have low specificity.

The common presenting symptoms and their frequencies are summarized in table 2.

Since lower limb DVT is the cause of PE in the majority of cases, it is prudent to look for features of DVT, namely, local pain, tenderness, redness and warmth. Unfortunately, these signs are also nonspecific and may even be misleading at times.

| Table 2: Prevalence of Symptoms and Signs in Patients with Suspected Pulmonary Embolism According to Final Diagnosis[17,19,20] | |
| --- | --- |
| **Symptoms** | **Percentage (%)** |
| Dyspnea | 80 |
| Chest pain (pleuritic) | 52 |
| Chest pain (substernal) | 12 |
| Cough | 37 |
| Leg pain | 26 |
| Syncope | 19 |
| Hemoptysis | 11 |
| **Signs** | **Percentage (%)** |
| Tachypnea | 70 |
| Tachycardia | 26 |
| Loud P2 | 23 |
| Signs of deep vein thrombosis cyanosis | 15 |
| Cyanosis | 11 |
| Fever | 7 |

# DIAGNOSIS

The diagnosis of PE requires the integration of a careful history and physical examination with laboratory testing and appropriate imaging modalities.

## Routine and Ancillary Investigations

A chest radiograph is usually the first investigation ordered for a patient presenting with symptoms of PE, followed by electrocardiogram (ECG). Routine investigations like chest X-ray, ECG and two-dimensional echocardiography (2D-Echo) are of limited value in the diagnosis of PE.

Chest radiographic abnormalities are commonly seen in patients with PE; however, they are not helpful diagnostically, because they are nonspecific. ECG may show sinus tachycardia and atrial arrhythmia. In particular, new-onset atrial flutter should increase suspicion of acute PE.[21]

Echocardiography is best used in suspected or proven acute PE to assess the impact of acute PE on right ventricular function. A regional pattern of right ventricular dysfunction, with akinesia of the mid free wall and right ventricular free wall but normal apical contractility, i.e., McConnell's sign; acute right ventricular infarction may also cause a similar appearance. Rarely, echocardiogram may identify emboli in-transit in the right atrium and if noted before lung imaging, may obviate the need for the same.

Arterial blood gas analysis often demonstrates hypoxemia and hypocapnia, but it may also be normal, especially in younger patients without cardiopulmonary disease.[20] In the setting of a normal or near normal chest radiograph and significant unexplained hypoxemia, PE should be considered.

D-dimers are formed as a result of fibrin degradation and rise with intravascular coagulation. The levels in plasma reflect the fibrinolytic activity on pre-existing thrombi and not necessarily the rate of thrombus formation itself. D-dimer tests are nonspecific and may be elevated in various conditions like cancer, recent surgery, renal insufficiency, pregnancy, and several other conditions.[22,23] Therefore in hospitalized patients, elevated D-dimer is a common finding.

D-dimer tests have low specificity and positive predictive value and, therefore, elevated D-dimers cannot be used for the confirmation of diagnosis of PE nor a normal D-dimer test be used to overrule the clinical judgment of a physician in suspecting and performing further investigations for PE in patients with high clinical probability.[15,24] However, the test has a high negative predictive value and reliably excludes PE in patients with low or intermediate clinical probability.[12]

Serum troponin may be elevated in acute PE, indicating right ventricular ischemia or microinfarction.[25] Brain natriuretic peptide (BNP) levels may also be elevated in acute PE because of right ventricular dilation. This may serve as a clue to the diagnosis, but is nonspecific.

## Diagnostic Imaging for Suspected Pulmonary Embolism

### Deep Venous Thrombosis Testing

Compression ultrasonography (CUS) is used as an indirect method for diagnosing PE. CUS has a sensitivity over 90% for proximal DVT and a specificity of about 95%.[26,27] It shows DVT in 30–50% of patients with PE,[26,27] and finding a proximal DVT in patients suspected of PE is sufficient to warrant anticoagulant treatment without further testing.[15] The only validated diagnostic criterion for DVT is incomplete compressibility of the vein, which indicates the presence of a clot, whereas flow criteria are unreliable.[15] When CUS is positive in patients with contraindications to contrast dye and/or irradiation, CT can be avoided.[15]

### Radioisotope Ventilation-perfusion Scan

Ventilation-perfusion scintigraphy (V/Q scan) is a well-established diagnostic test for suspected PE. It is noninvasive and safe to use; barring few allergic reactions that have been described. The ventilation and perfusion phases of a V/Q lung scan are performed together and may include a chest X-ray for comparison or to look for other causes of lung disease. A defect in the perfusion images requires a mismatched ventilation defect to be indicative of PE.

Diagnostic accuracy of the V/Q scan is greatest when the test is combined with clinical probability:[28]

- Patients with high clinical probability of PE and a high-probability V/Q scan had a 95% likelihood of having PE
- Patients with low clinical probability of PE and a low-probability V/Q scan had only a 4% likelihood of having PE
- A normal V/Q scan virtually excludes PE
- Strong clinical suspicion of PE in the presence of a nondiagnostic V/Q scan should lead to further evaluation [computed tomography (CT) angiography, pulmonary angiography or lower limb DVT studies].

### Computed Tomography Pulmonary Arteriography

Computed tomography pulmonary arteriography (CTPA) has become the most commonly used diagnostic modality for patients with suspected PE (Figures 3 and 4). One of the most commonly cited benefits of CTPA is its ability to detect alternative pulmonary abnormalities that may explain the patient's clinical presentation.[29,30] With spiral CT, the location and the magnitude of the thrombus are demonstrated and both mediastinal and parenchymal structures are evaluated which may provide important alternate or additional diagnoses.

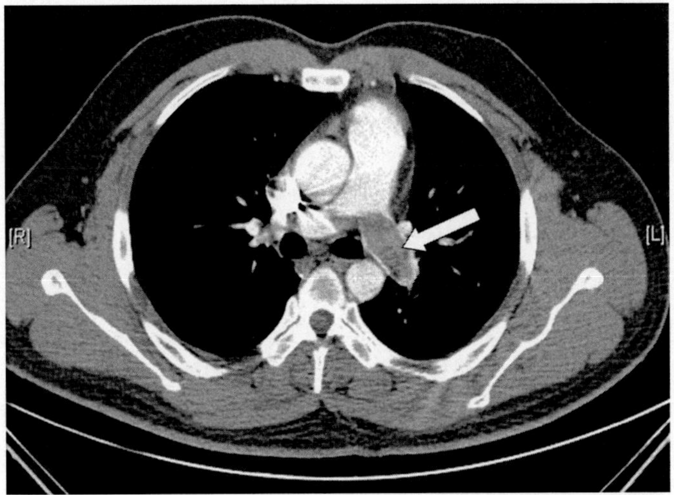

**Figure 3:** Computed tomography angiography showing a massive pulmonary embolism.

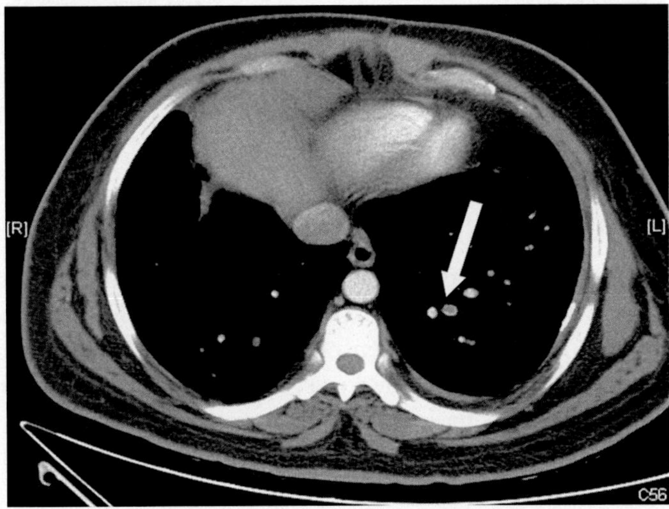

**Figure 4:** Thrombus in a smaller branch of pulmonary artery.

Early studies comparing conventional single-slice spiral CT with selective pulmonary arteriography demonstrated high accuracy of spiral CT for detecting PE from the main pulmonary artery to the segmental arterial level[31,32] but had concluded that subsegmental emboli may be missed. Limitations for the inability to make a reliable diagnosis of small peripheral emboli, with a reported miss rate of up to 30% with single-slice spiral CT, had prevented the unanimous embrace of single-slice spiral CT as the standard of reference for imaging PE.[33]

The advent of the multidetector CT (MDCT) angiography largely overcame the limitations with regards to the accuracy of spiral CT. The use of MDCT angiography has led to decreased section thickness, reduced scanning times, and markedly improved visualization of segmental and subsegmental vessels.[34] With improved diagnosis of small peripheral emboli, MDCT has emerged as a preferred modality for imaging patients with suspected acute PE. When either single-detector or MDCT arteriography suggests acute PE, treatment is nearly always mandated; false positive CT angiographic studies appear to be unusual. According to the Prospective Investigation of Pulmonary Embolism Diagnosis II (PIOPED II) study,[35] the sensitivity of MDCT was 83% and the specificity was 96%. Thus, new generation MDCT is now a challenge to catheter pulmonary angiography, the gold standard, for the accurate detection of PE.[33] Nonetheless, it is prudent to consider pulmonary angiography in cases of high clinical suspicion, even if CT arteriography is negative.

The combination of CT arteriography and CT venography (for detection of DVT) has been assessed in some trials.[28,36] Most recently, the PIOPED II trial compared the use of MDCT arteriography alone with its use in combination with CT venography for detecting suspected acute PE.[28] The sensitivity of spiral CT arteriography alone was 83%, whereas the combination of CT arteriography and CT venography increased the sensitivity to 90%, suggesting that a combined approach might facilitate clinical management, particularly for the treatment of in-patients with complex cases.

### Pulmonary Angiography

Pulmonary angiography is still the gold standard investigation for the confirmation of PE.[37] It is an invasive procedure with potential risks and is, therefore, performed very infrequently. It is indicated when cardiovascular collapse and hypotension are present for quick definitive diagnosis, and when other investigations are inconclusive. The features indicating the presence of an embolus include intraluminal filling defect and abrupt vascular cut-off in pulmonary arteries. Fatal complications occur in 0.5–1.3% of the procedures and minor complications in 2% of patients.[18]

### Clinical Probability

In a patient with suspected PE, clinical probability assessment is considered to be an essential step. The clinical pretest probability can be determined by taking into account patient's clinical history, risk factors for VTE, clinical signs, and the laboratory tests. The implicit evaluation of pretest probability was demonstrated to be relatively accurate in the PIOPED study.[28] Various clinical prediction rules are available for the diagnosis of PE, but the most widely used and validated in diagnostic studies are (i) the Wells score[38] and (ii) the Geneva score.[39] The revised Geneva score proposed in 2006 is independent of the clinical judgment, chest radiographs and arterial blood gas analysis.[40]

Using one of the clinical prediction rules,[38,40] the prevalence of confirmed PE is found to be 10% in low probability category, 30% in moderate category and 70% in high probability category.[41] Various combinations using clinical probability scores, D-dimer assays, lower limb imaging, V/Q lung scintigraphy and spiral CT have been evaluated in various studies to formulate diagnostic algorithms and for risk stratifications in patients with suspected PE.

## MANAGEMENT

### General Management

Generally, when PE is diagnosed, inpatient therapy with initial bed rest for 24–48 hours is recommended. Analgesia should be given to patients with severe pleuritic pain, but opiates should be avoided in patients with incipient cardiovascular collapse since they cause vasodilatation. Hypoxemia should be treated with high percentage inspired oxygen, severe hypoxia may require ventilation. In hypotensive patients, colloid should be administered while monitoring central venous pressure and the right atrial pressure should be maintained high (15–20 mmHg) to ensure maximal right ventricular filling. Use of inotropic agents may be required to provide circulatory support. Diuretics and vasodilators are not indicated.[18]

### Specific Treatment

From the point of view of therapy, patients suffering from PE can be classified into one of the following subsets:[42]

- Stable pulmonary embolism: normotensive patients [when systolic BP (SBP) ≥90 mmHg] with no evidence of right ventricular dysfunction
- Submassive pulmonary embolism: normotensive patients (SBP ≥90 mmHg) with evidence of right ventricular dysfunction
- Massive pulmonary embolism: patient is hypotensive in cardiogenic shock (SBP <90 mmHg) or cardiac arrest or there is fall in SBP by greater than 40 mmHg for at least 15 minutes.

Anticoagulation is the mainstay of treatment for acute PE. Stable PE can be managed in hospital or on an outpatient basis with anticoagulation either with unfractionated heparin (UFH) or low molecular weight heparin (LMWH) or factor Xa inhibitor—fondaparinux. Massive and submassive PE carry high mortality; modalities to achieve early reperfusion of the pulmonary arteries may be lifesaving by reversing the right ventricular dysfunction. Various options available are thrombolysis, surgical embolectomy, and percutaneous catheter embolectomy.

## Anticoagulant Therapy

Anticoagulant treatment plays a critical role in the management of patients with PE and is required universally regardless of whether they have undergone reperfusion therapy for massive and submassive PE. Anticoagulants help in preventing formation of new thrombus, death and recurrent events with an acceptable rate of bleeding complications. The agents that are used for anticoagulation are as follows:

1. *Unfractionated heparin*: unfractionated heparin acts by binding to antithrombin and catalyzing the inactivation of thrombin factor Xa and other clotting factors. Besides, it also binds with other plasma proteins resulting in unpredictable pharmacokinetic and pharmacodynamic properties which can lead to nonhemorrhagic side effects such as heparin-induced thrombocytopenia (HIT) and osteoporosis. Since the anticoagulant effect of UFH which can be rapidly reversed, it is the agent of choice for patients with PE who are at high risk of bleeding. There are several regimens of heparin therapy.[43]

   For the intravenous regimen, the bolus dose followed by continuous infusion is titrated to a target activated partial thromboplastin time (APTT) of 1.5–2.5 times of control (approximately 60–80 seconds). The first measurement of APTT should be performed 4–6 hours after starting treatment to ensure adequate anticoagulation and repeated 3 hours after every change of dose and subsequently at least daily after target therapeutic dose is reached. Dosing based on patient's body weight is preferable to a standard regimen, since it causes fewer fluctuations in APTT and achieves a therapeutic level more quickly with a shorter warfarin overlap. Subcutaneous heparin does not require frequent monitoring, is found to be as safe and effective as weight-adjusted LMWH.[43]

   The important complications associated with heparin are bleeding, immune-mediated platelet activation leading to HIT and osteoporosis. Sometimes, dermatological side effects such as necrosis, alopecia, and hypersensitivity are encountered. HIT is usually seen 4–14 days after heparin therapy can lead to major bleeding and thrombotic complications. HIT does not respond to platelet transfusion and heparin must be stopped. HIT may respond to plasmapheresis.

2. *Low molecular weight heparin*: low molecular weight heparins are derived from UFH by chemical or enzymatic depolymerization. LMWHs should be given with care in patients with renal failure. Intravenous UFH may be the preferred mode of initial anticoagulation for patients with severe renal impairment

(creatinine clearance <30 mL/minute), and with severe risk of bleeding. The American College of Chest Physicians consensus statement on VTE recommends subcutaneous LMWH over standard, UFH.[44] The advantages of LMWH over UFH are tabulated. Therefore, in most cases of acute PE, LMWH should be given subcutaneously at weight-adjusted doses without monitoring.[15]

3. *Fondaparinux*: fondaparinux is a synthetic polysaccharide with anti-Xa activity. It has been shown to be as effective as heparin and is not associated with HIT. Dosage is required once daily and is weight related. It is contraindicated in severe renal failure (creatinine clearance <30 mL/minute).

Rapid anticoagulation can be achieved with parenteral anticoagulants such as intravenous UFH, fixed dose subcutaneous UFH, subcutaneous LMWH or subcutaneous fondaparinux. Anticoagulation should be initiated without delay in patients with confirmed PE and in those with a high or intermediate clinical probability of PE, while awaiting definitive diagnostic confirmation (in the absence of any contraindication).[15]

### Long-term Anticoagulation

Long-term anticoagulation to prevent clot recurrence is usually achieved by oral vitamin K antagonists (VKAs) like warfarin or acenocoumarol. However, it should be initiated once PE has been reliably confirmed.

If warfarin is used, a starting dose of 5 mg or 7.5 mg is preferred over higher doses. Studies performed in hospitalized patients showed that starting warfarin at a dose of 5 mg was associated with less excessive anticoagulation compared with 10 mg, although therapeutic INR (>1.9) was achieved 1.4 days sooner in 10 mg protocol.[45] Clot recurrence, bleeding events and morbidity profiles did not differ in two groups. Taken together, these data suggest that warfarin can usually be started at a dose of 10 mg in younger patients (<60 years) and in otherwise healthy outpatients, and at a dose of 5 mg in older patients and in those who are hospitalized. Subsequent doses should be adjusted to maintain the INR at a target of 2.5 (range 2.0–3.0).[15] The recommended dosage schedules for initiation of warfarin I generally with 5 mg/day.[46]

### Monitoring of Oral Anticoagulants

In patients beginning VKA therapy, INR should be monitored after the initial two or three doses of oral anticoagulation therapy and dose adjustment is made based on this till the target INR is reached. For patients who are receiving a stable dose of oral anticoagulants, monitoring should be done at an interval of no longer than every 4 weeks.[47]

### Newer Oral Anticoagulants

Dabigatran etexilate (direct thrombin inhibitor, IIa), rivaroxaban, and apixaban (direct coagulation factor Xa inhibitor) are the Food and Drug Administration (FDA)-approved newer oral anticoagulants (NOACs) for clinical use in countries like the United States of America and Canada. Several phase III clinical trials have proved their safety and efficacy in different clinical situations.[48,49]

These drugs have been approved by FDA, European Medicines Agency (EMA), and Canada's Health Products and Food branch for following indications:

- Prevention of stroke and systemic embolism in adult patients with nonvalvular atrial fibrillation (AF)
- Primary prevention of VTE in adult patients who have undergone elective total hip arthroplasty (THA) or total knee arthroplasty (TKA).

Newer oral anticoagulants have the potential to overcome the short comings of VKAs. These can be administered in fixed doses (Table 3) without need for close lab monitoring with no significant food-drug interactions. However, they are costly and lack specific antidotes as well as long-term safety data. Newer studies underway are likely to pave the way for more widespread use of NOACs in clinical practice.

### Duration of Anticoagulation Therapy

Duration of anticoagulant treatment in a particular patient should be ascertained depending on the risk-benefit assessment between the estimated risk of recurrence after treatment discontinuation and the risk of bleeding complications while on treatment. When there are transient risk factors for VTE, such as the postoperative period, recurrence during and after treatment is unusual. Recurrent embolism in the absence of a recurrent or new risk factor should be treated with long-term anticoagulation. In patients with persisting underlying risk factors, such as deficiency of antithrombin III, protein C, or protein S, the anticoagulation is usually prolonged to several years, possibly lifelong. Table 4 summarizes the recommendations on the duration of anticoagulation.[15]

| Table 3: Recommended Dosage of Newer Oral Anticoagulants (USA)[50] | | | |
|---|---|---|---|
| **Drug** | **Stroke prevention in nonvalvular AF** | **Postoperative thromboprophylaxis** | **DVT/PE** |
| Dabigatran* | 150 mg BD | – | – |
| Rivaroxaban* | 20 mg OD | 10 mg OD for 14 days for TKA<br>10 mg OD for 35 days for THR | 15 mg BD for 3 weeks followed by 20 mg OD |
| Apixaban* | 5 mg BD | – | – |

*Dose needs to be adjusted in renal insufficiency according to creatinine clearance.

AF, atrial fibrillation; BD, twice a day; OD, once a day; TKA, total knee arthroplasty; THR, total hip arthroplasty.

| Table 4: Recommendations for Duration of Anticoagulation[15] | |
| --- | --- |
| **Thromboembolism** | **Duration** |
| PE secondary to a transient (reversible) risk factor | 3 months |
| Unprovoked PE | At least 3 months |
| First episode of unprovoked PE and low risk of bleeding, and in whom stable anticoagulation can be achieved | May be considered for long-term anticoagulation |
| Second episode of unprovoked PE | Long-term anticoagulation |
| PE and cancer | LMWH should be considered for the first 3–6 months. After this period, anticoagulant therapy with VKA or LMWH should be continued indefinitely or until the cancer is cured |

PE, pulmonary embolism; LMWH, low molecular weight heparin; VKA, vitamin K antagonist.

There is evidence to suggest that D-dimer levels may help guide decisions about the duration of therapy; persistently elevated levels appear to be associated with an increased recurrence rate.[51] Long-term treatment of thrombosis with the LMWH dalteparin, as compared with warfarin, in patients with cancer has been shown to be associated with fewer thromboembolic recurrences.[52]

## Thrombolytic Therapy

Thrombolytic therapy is recommended as the first-line treatment for patients with massive PE (hemodynamic compromise/imminent cardiac arrest). Thrombolytic therapy should be instituted at the earliest in such patients provided there are no contraindications pertaining to risk of bleeding (Table 5). The therapy not

| Table 5: Contraindications for Thrombolytic Therapy[15] | |
| --- | --- |
| **Absolute** | **Relative** |
| • Hemorrhagic stroke or stroke of unknown origin at anytime | • Transient ischemic attack in preceding 6 months |
| • Ischemic stroke in preceding 6 months | • Oral anticoagulant therapy |
| • Central nervous system damage or neoplasm | • Pregnancy or within 1-week postpartum |
| • Recent major trauma/surgery/head injury (with in preceding 3 weeks) | • Noncompressible punctures |
| • Gastrointestinal bleeding within the last month | • Traumatic resuscitation |
| • Known active bleeding | • Refractory hypertension (systolic blood pressure >180 mmHg) |
| | • Advanced liver disease |
| | • Infective endocarditis |
| | • Active peptic ulcer |

only helps in achieving rapid resolution of PE but also rapid hemodynamic improvement. It has no role in the management of hemodynamically stable patients, except perhaps in the subgroup of patients with submassive PE (right ventricular dysfunction but normal systemic arterial pressure), in which there is some evidence for its efficacy. Thrombolytic treatment is most effective when administered soon after the onset of PE, but benefit may extend for up to 14 days from the onset of symptoms.[18] While thrombolysis may be lifesaving in massive and submassive PE, the extent of long-term survival and reduction in mortality at 90 days remains unclear.

Drawbacks of thrombolytic therapy are high cost, risk of severe, and often fatal bleeding and allergic reactions (specifically to streptokinase).

## Inferior Vena Caval Filters

Inferior vena caval (IVC) filter devices placed in the IVC protect the pulmonary circulation from emboli. The routine use of IVC filters in patients with PE is not recommended, since they are associated with complications and late sequelae, including recurrent DVT episodes and development of the post-thrombotic syndrome. The two main indications for the use of filters are: (i) absolute contraindications to anticoagulation and (ii) high risk of VTE recurrence.

## Surgical Management

### Surgical Embolectomy

Surgical embolectomy has been reserved for a selective group of patients who have massive PE with hemodynamic instability requiring cardiopulmonary resuscitation or who have failed thrombolytic therapy or have contraindications to its use. It may also be performed in patients with patent foramen ovale and intracardiac thrombi.[50] However, this procedure should be attempted only in centers with the necessary skills and experience.

### Catheter Embolectomy

Catheter-based mechanical pulmonary embolectomy, local intraembolic thrombolytic therapy, or both may be considered as alternatives to surgical embolectomy for the same indications.[53]

### Risk Stratification in Acute Pulmonary Embolism

Risk stratification of PE has gained importance, to ensure that the appropriate management is instituted. There has been increasing interest in identifying low-risk patients with PE who could be offered outpatient treatment or a short hospital stay. A clinical score for predicting early mortality in patients with PE has recently been described by Aujesky[53] and associates and has been validated in other cohorts.

Another challenge lies with regard to the management of a patient who is not hemodynamically compromised, but in whom there appears to be a high risk of decompensation. Patients with "submassive PE" fall into this category.

A number of studies offer compelling arguments that right ventricular dysfunction is an important marker for mortality.[54] The factors that may support a more aggressive approach in this setting which could have more extreme right ventricular dysfunction and may reveal ECG abnormalities, such as T-wave inversion or a pseudoinfarction pattern (Qr), in the anterior precordial leads. These findings suggests right ventricular dilation and dysfunction, which can be integrated into risk stratification decisions.[55]

Recent data suggest that mortality due to acute PE is higher in the setting of residual deep venous thrombosis, and so the evaluation of the legs as part of the risk stratification protocol in acute PE should be considered.[56]

The role of biomarkers in risk stratification has shown some promise. High levels of BNP, pro-BNP, and cardiac troponins (both T and I) have been associated with a greater risk of death in patients with PE. Any elevation in troponin level confers a fivefold increase in short-term mortality.[57]

## CONCLUSION

Pulmonary venous thromboembolism is a potentially fatal disorder that is unsuspected and undiagnosed in several hospitalized patients. The clinical presentation of PE is variable and at times nonspecific, making the diagnosis challenging. However, a high index of clinical suspicion is required in the setting of appropriate risk factors to select the patients that require evaluation for PE; to ensure early diagnosis, risk stratification, and appropriate management. The use of multidetector CTPA has significantly improved the diagnostic sensitivity for PE and is the most widely confirmatory test. The invasive gold standard test—pulmonary angiography—is rarely performed in clinical practice. Early institution of treatment helps in reducing the morbidity as well as mortality. Anticoagulation is the back bone of treatment. Anticoagulant treatment is initiated preferably with low molecular weight heparins and long-term anticoagulation treatment is given using conventional oral VKA. However, newer oral anticoagulants have the potential to overcome the short comings of VKAs and may become the standard of care in the future.

### Editor's Comment

*Pulmonary embolism continues to be often missed in the intensive care unit (ICU) and is associated with a significant morbidity and mortality. The use of ultrasound in the ICU has made a great difference in the diagnosis and severity assessment in these patients. Lower limb screening ultrasound should be done in the ICU almost every day to look for deep vein thrombosis (DVT). Most intensivists need to be well versed with using ultrasound in ICU patients, as this will help in the early diagnosis of DVT and pulmonary embolism besides other things. Computed tomography pulmonary angiography has become the diagnostic modality of choice for pulmonary embolism. They have a very high sensitivity and specificity and only small subsegmental emboli can be missed. Once diagnosed, the treatment strategy depends upon the severity of the pulmonary embolism. If these are features of hemodynamic instability or signs of right ventricular dysfunction, thrombolytic therapy should be considered. Most studies now show that longer anticoagulation even in patients who have a reversible factor is preferable, as there is a risk if recurrence of the thrombus. Newer oral anticoagulants are now available and they need no monitoring unlike the older oral anticoagulants.*

**Randeep Guleria**

## REFERENCES


1. Lilienfeld DE. Decreasing mortality from pulmonary embolism in the United States, 1979-1996. *Int J Epidemiol.* 2000;29:465-9.
2. Moser KM, Fedullo PF, LitteJohn JK, Crawford R. Frequent asymptomatic pulmonary embolism in patients with deep venous thrombosis. *JAMA.* 1994;271:223-5.
3. Dalen JE. Pulmonary embolism: what have we learned since Virchow? Natural history, pathophysiology, and diagnosis. *Chest.* 2002;122:1440-56.
4. Kearon C. Natural history of venous thromboembolism. *Circulation.* 2003;107(23 Suppl 1):I22-30.
5. Murin S, Romano PS, White RH. Comparison of outcomes after hospitalization for deep venous thrombosis or pulmonary embolism. *Thromb Haemost.* 2002;88:407-14.
6. Stein PD, Kayali F, Olson RE. Estimated case fatality rate of pulmonary embolism, 1979 to 1998. *Am J Cardiol.* 2004;93:1197-9.
7. Oger E. Incidence of venous thromboembolism: a community-based study in Western France. EPI-GETBP Study Group. Groupe d'Etude de la Thrombose de Bretagne Occidentale. *Thromb Haemost.* 2000;83:657-60.
8. Silverstein MD, Heit JA, Mohr DN, Petterson TM, O'Fallon WM, Melton LJ 3rd. Trends in the incidence of deep vein thrombosis and pulmonary embolism: a 25-year population-based study. *Arch Intern Med.* 1998;158:585-93.
9. Cohen AT, Agnelli G, Anderson FA, Arcelus JI, Bergqvist D, Brecht JG, et al. Venous thromboembolism (VTE) in Europe. The number of VTE events and associated morbidity and mortality. *Thromb Haemost.* 2007;98:756-64.
10. Bonderman D, Wilkens H, Wakounig S, Schäfers HJ, Jansa P, Lindner J, et al. Risk factors for chronic thromboembolic pulmonary hypertension. *Eur Respir J.* 2009;33:325-31.
11. Condliffe R, Kiely DG, Gibbs JS, Corris PA, Peacock AJ, Jenkins DP, et al. Prognostic and aetiological factors in chronic thromboembolic pulmonary hypertension. *Eur Respir J.* 2009;33:332-8.

12. British Thoracic Society Standards of Care Committee Pulmonary Embolism Guideline Development Group. British Thoracic Society guidelines for the management of suspected acute pulmonary embolism. *Thorax.* 2003;58:470-83.

13. Pomp ER, Lenselink AM, Rosendaal FR, Doggen CJ. Pregnancy, the postpartum period and prothrombotic defects: risk of venous thrombosis in the MEGA study. *J Thromb Haemost.* 2008;6:632-7.

14. Vandenbroucke JP, Rosing J, Bloemenkamp KW, Middeldorp S, Helmerhorst FM, Bouma BN, et al. Oral contraceptives and the risk of venous thrombosis. *N Engl J Med.* 2001;344:1527-35.

15. Torbicki A, Perrier A, Konstantinides S, Agnelli G, Galiè N, Pruszczyk P, et al. Guidelines on the diagnosis and management of acute pulmonary embolism: the Task Force for the Diagnosis and Management of Acute Pulmonary Embolism of the European Society of Cardiology (ESC). *Eur Heart J.* 2008;29:2276-315.

16. Wells PS, Ginsberg JS, Anderson DR, Kearon C, Gent M, Turpie AG, et al. Use of a clinical model for safe management of patients with suspected pulmonary embolism. *Ann Intern Med.* 1998;129:997-1005.

17. Miniati M, Prediletto R, Formichi B, Marini C, Di Ricco G, Tonelli L, et al. Accuracy of clinical assessment in the diagnosis of pulmonary embolism. *Am J Respir Crit Care Med.* 1999;159:864-71.

18. Christopher DJ, Ruffin RE. Pulmonary embolism. In: Ratnaike RN (Ed). Essential Guide to Geriatric Practice. USA: McGraw-Hill; 2001.

19. Stein PD, Saltzman HA, Weg JG. Clinical characteristics of patients with acute pulmonary embolism. *Am J Cardiol.* 1991;68:1723-4.

20. Stein PD, Terrin ML, Hales CA, Palevsky HI, Saltzman HA, Thompson BT, et al. Clinical, laboratory, roentgenographic, and electrocardiographic findings in patients with Pulmonary embolism and no pre-existing cardiac or pulmonary disease. *Chest.* 1991;100(3):598-603.

21. Johson JC, Flowers NC, Horan LG. Unexplained atrial flutter: a frequent herald of pulmonary embolism. *Chest.* 1971;60:29-34.

22. Miron MJ, Perrier A, Bounameaux H, de Moerloose P, Slosman DO, Didier D, et al. Contribution of noninvasive evaluation to the diagnosis of pulmonary embolism in hospitalized patients. *Eur Respir J.* 1999;13:1365-70.

23. Ghirardini G, Battioni M, Bertellini C, Colombini R, Colla R, Rossi G. D-dimer after delivery in uncomplicated pregnancies. *Clin Exp Obstet Gynecol.* 1999;26:211-2.

24. Di Nisio M, Squizzato A, Rutjes AW, Büller HR, Zwinderman AH, Bossuyt PM. Diagnostic accuracy of D-dimer test for exclusion of venous thromboembolism: a systematic review. *J Thromb Haemost.* 2007;5:296-304.

25. Scridon T, Scridon C, Skali H, Alvarez A, Goldhaber SZ, Solomon SD. Prognostic significance of troponin elevation and right ventricular enlargement in acute pulmonary embolism. *Am J Cardiol.* 2005;96:303-5.

26. Kearon C, Ginsberg JS, Hirsh J. The role of venous ultrasonography in the diagnosis of suspected deep venous thrombosis and pulmonary embolism. *Ann Intern Med.* 1998;129:1044-9.

27. Perrier A, Bounameaux H. Ultrasonography of leg veins in patients suspected of having pulmonary embolism. *Ann Intern Med.* 1998;128:243-5.

28. PIOPED Investigators. Value of the ventilation/perfusion scan in acute pulmonary embolism. Results of the prospective investigation of pulmonary embolism diagnosis (PIOPED). *JAMA.* 1990;263:2753-9.

29. Kim, KI, Muller, NL, Mayo, JR. Clinically suspected pulmonary embolism: utility of spiral CT. *Radiology.* 1999;210:693-7.

30. Garg K, Sieler H, Welsh CH, Johnston RJ, Russ PD. Clinical validity of helical CT being interpreted as negative for pulmonary embolism: implications for patient treatment. *AJR Am J Roentgenol.* 1999;172:1627-31.

31. Remy-Jardin M, Remy J, Deschildre F, Artaud D, Beregi JP, Hossein-Foucher C, et al. Diagnosis of pulmonary embolism with spiral CT: comparison with pulmonary angiography and scintigraphy. *Radiology.* 1996;200:699-706.

32. Teigen CL, Maus TP, Sheedy PF 2nd, Stanson AW, Johnson CM, Breen JF, et al. Pulmonary embolism: diagnosis with contrast-enhanced electron-beam CT and comparison with pulmonary angiography. *Radiology.* 1995;194:313-9.

33. Schoepf UJ, Goldhaber SZ, Costello P. Spiral computed tomography for acute pulmonary embolism. *Circulation.* 2004;109:2160-7.

34. Drucker EA, Rivitz SM, Shepard JA, Boiselle PM, Trotman-Dickenson B, Welch TJ, et al. Acute pulmonary embolism: assessment of helical CT for diagnosis. *Radiology.* 1998;209:235-41.

35. Stein PD, Fowler SE, Goodman LR, Gottschalk A, Hales CA, Hull RD, et al. Multidetector computed tomography for acute pulmonary embolism. *N Engl J Med.* 2006;354(22):2317-27.

36. Loud PA, Katz DS, Bruce DA, Klippenstein DL, Grossman ZD. Deep venous thrombosis with suspected pulmonary embolism: detection with combined CT venography and pulmonary angiography. *Radiology.* 2001;219:498-502.

37. Gupta S, Gupta BM. Acute pulmonary embolism advances in treatment. *J Assoc Physicians India.* 2008;56: 185-91.

38. Wells PS, Anderson DR, Rodger M, Ginsberg JS, Kearon C, Gent M, et al. Derivation of a simple clinical model to categorize patients probability of pulmonary embolism: increasing the models utility with the SimpliRED D-dimer. *Thromb Haemost.* 2000;83:416-20.

39. Wicki J, Perneger TV, Junod AF, Bounameaux H, Perrier A. Assessing clinical probability of pulmonary embolism in the emergency ward: a simple score. *Arch Intern Med.* 2001;161:92-7.

40. Le Gal G, Righini M, Roy PM, Sanchez O, Aujesky D, Bounameaux H, et al. Prediction of pulmonary embolism in the emergency department: the revised Geneva score. *Ann Intern Med.* 2006;144:165-71.

41. Klok FA, Kruisman E, Spaan J, Nijkeuter M, Righini M, Aujesky D, et al. Comparison of the revised Geneva score with the Wells rule for assessing clinical probability of pulmonary embolism. *J Thromb Haemost.* 2008;6:40-4.

42. Piazza G, Goldhaber SZ. Acute pulmonary embolism: part II: treatment and prophylaxis. *Circulation.* 2006;114:e42-7.

43. Kearon C, Ginsberg JS, Julian JA, Douketis J, Solymoss S, Ockelford P, et al. Comparison of fixed-dose weight-adjusted unfractionated heparin and low-molecular-weight heparin for acute treatment of venous thromboembolism. *JAMA.* 2006;296:935-42.

44. Kearon C, Kahn SR, Agnelli G, Goldhaber S, Raskob GE, Comerota AJ, et al. Antithrombotic therapy for venous thromboembolic disease: American College of Chest Physicians Evidence-based Clinical Practice Guidelines (8th edition). *Chest.* 2008;133:454S-545S.

45. Kovacs MJ, Rodger MA, Anderson DR, Morrow B, Kells G, Kovacs J. Comparison of 10-mg and 5-mg warfarin initiation nomograms together with low-molecular-weight heparin for outpatient treatment of acute venous thromboembolism. A randomized, double-blind, controlled trial. *Annals Intern Med.* 2003;138:714-9.

46. Crowther MA, Harrison L, Hirsh J. Reply: warfarin: less may be better. *Ann Intern Med.* 1997:127:333.

47. Ansell J, Hirsh J, Hylek E, Jacobson A, Crowther M, Palareti G, et al. Pharmacology and management of the vitamin K antagonists. American College of Chest Physicians Evidence-based Clinical Practice Guidelines (8th edition). *Chest.* 2008;133:160S-98S.

48. Guyatt GH, Akl EA, Crowther M, Schünemann HJ, Gutterman DD, Zelman Lewis S, et al. Introduction to the 9th edition: Antithrombotic therapy and prevention of Thrombosis, 9th ed: American College of Chest Physicians Evidence-Based Clinical Practice Guidelines. *Chest.* 2012;141(2 Suppl):48S-52S.

49. Gonsalves WI, Pruthi RK, Patnaik MM. The new oral anticoagulants in clinical practice. *Mayo Clin Proc.* 2013;88(5):495-511.

50. Tapson VF, Gurbel PA, Witty LA, Pieper KS, Stack RS. Pharmacomechanical thrombolysis of experimental pulmonary emboli. Rapid low-dose intraembolic therapy. *Chest.* 1994;106:1558-62.

51. Aujesky D, Obrosky DS, Stone RA, Auble TE, Perrier A, Cornuz J, et al. Derivation and validation of a prognostic model for pulmonary embolism. *Am J Respir Crit Care Med.* 2005;172:1041-6.

52. Yalamanchili K, Fleisher AG, Lehrman SG, Axelrod HI, Lafaro RJ, Sarabu MR, et al. Open pulmonary embolectomy for treatment of major pulmonary embolism. *Ann Thorac Surg.* 2004;77:819-23.

53. Aujesky D, Perrier A, Roy PM, Stone RA, Cornuz J, Meyer G, et al. Validation of a clinical prognostic model to identify low-risk patients with pulmonary embolism. *J Intern Med.* 2007;261:597-604.

54. Ribeiro A, Lindmarker P, Juhlin-Dannfelt A, Johnsson H, Jorfeldt L. Echocardiography Doppler in pulmonary embolism: right ventricular dysfunction as a predictor of mortality rate. *Am Heart J.* 1997;134:479-87.

55. Pruszczyk P, Bochowicz A, Torbicki A, Szulc M, Kurzyna M, Fijałkowska A, et al. Cardiac troponin T monitoring identifies high-risk group of normotensive patients with acute pulmonary embolism. *Chest.* 2003;123:1947-52.

56. Jiménez D, Aujesky D, Díaz G, Monreal M, Otero R, Martí D, et al. Prognostic significance of deep vein thrombosis in patients presenting with acute symptomatic pulmonary embolism. *Am J Respir Crit Care Med.* 2010;181:983-91.

57. Becattini C, Vedovati MC, Agnelli G. Prognostic value of troponins in acute pulmonary embolism: a meta-analysis. *Circulation.* 2007;116:427-33.

World Clin Pulm Crit Care Med. 2016;4(1):101-22.

# Critical Care in Case of Poisoning

[1]Inderpaul S Sehgal MD DNB DM, [2,]*Dhruva Chaudhry MD DNB DM FICP FICCM

[1]Department of Pulmonary Medicine, Postgraduate Institute of Medical Education and Research
Chandigarh, India
[2]Department of Pulmonary and Critical Care Medicine
Pt. BD Sharma Post Graduate Institute of Medical Sciences, Rohtak, Haryana, India

## *ABSTRACT*

Accidental or self-induced poisoning is medical emergency that needs high clinical suspicion and a systematic approach for early diagnosis and treatment. The management involves supportive care that includes securing of the airway, breathing, and circulation and decontamination to prevent further absorption of the offending poison or a drug. Poisoning presents with a myriad of clinical features and needs a syndromic approach (sympathomimetic, sympatholytic, cholinergic, or anticholinergic syndrome) to identify the offending agent. Once patient is stabilized an attempt to correctly identify the specific poisoning agent or drug should be made either by revisiting the clinical details and/or performing a toxicology screen on blood and or urine specimens. Once identified, specific antidote should be instituted to hasten the clinical recovery and prevent further organ damage due to the offending agent.

## INTRODUCTION

Acute poisoning is an important medical emergency needing admission in critical care units. A poisoning is an event where a living organism is exposed to a chemical that adversely affects the functioning of that organism.[1] The exposure of the toxin may be occupational, environmental, recreational, or medicinal and can occur from varied portals of entry, but predominantly from ingestion. A poison may affect the body in many ways. It may inhibit, or alter the normal cellular function, change normal organ function, or may change the normal uptake or transport of substances into or within the organism.[2]

*Corresponding author
*Email:* dhruvachaudhry@yahoo.co.in

The nature of poison varies in different parts of the world and in different parts of a country depending on the socioeconomic factors and cultural diversity.[3] Self-poisoning, including from pesticides, accounts for about one-third of the world's suicides. Official data from India probably underestimate the incidence of suicides. The proportion of all suicides with pesticides varies from 4% in the European region to over 50% in the Western Pacific region. It is the pattern of pesticide use and the toxicity of the products, not the quantity used, that influences the likelihood that they will be used in acts of fatal self-harm.[4] In general, accidental poisoning is more common in children, whereas suicidal poisoning is more common in young adults.[5]

It is important for the intensivists to know the pattern of poisoning in their area. Across India, pesticides [organophosphates (OPs) and organochlorine (OCL)] and fumicide (aluminum phosphide) are the commonest poisons used for self-harm in rural and semi-urban areas, whereas household products and drugs are commoner in metropolitan/city areas.[6] Epidemiological studies demonstrating the patterns of poisoning in critical care are scanty. It is believed that majority of cases of severe intoxication and deaths due to poisoning in critical care units across the country occurs due to pesticides and fumicides.[5-8]

The protean manifestations of intoxication mandate a higher index of suspicion to facilitate decision and immediate treatment, while the nature of the ingestion is confirmed. General supportive measures supersede all other considerations. For effective management of acutely poisoned victim, the following should be considered:

- Resuscitation and stabilization
- Establishing diagnosis of poisoning and drug overdose, including history, physical examination, use of toxicological screening tests including other common laboratory tests
- Prevention of further drug absorption, elimination of absorbed drugs, and antidotes
- Specific approaches for evaluation and treatment of commonly encountered drugs, toxins, and envenomation in the intensive care unit.

## RESUSCITATION AND STABILIZATION

Initial step is to identify and treat immediate life-threatening problems and revolves around pneumonic ABCD (Airway, Breathing, Circulation, Drugs, and Decontamination).

### Airway

Airway patency and stabilization must be established. In comatose patients, upper airway obstruction by the tongue may be treated initially with jaw thrust maneuver, followed by either placement of oral or nasal airway or an endotracheal tube. The choice of airway depends upon the level of sensorium, presence of protective reflexes, degree of respiratory depression and the initial response to pharmacological therapy.

## Breathing

It includes oxygenation and ventilation. In case of doubts regarding patient's ability to handle secretion or maintenance of spontaneous respirations, endotracheal intubation should be done immediately. Intubation allows administration of high concentration of supplemental oxygen in hypoxemic patients and assisted ventilation in patients with respiratory failure.

Hypoxemia should be corrected immediately to avoid anoxic damage to brain, myocardial ischemia, and cardiac arrhythmias. If the intubation is done solely for airway protection or to provide supplemental oxygen, then it must be connected to a T-piece. For patients with ventilatory failure, ventilation is achieved by mechanical ventilation.

## Circulation

After ensuring adequate airway patency, oxygenation, and ventilation, circulatory status of patient should be assessed. Circulatory manifestations of poisoning can range from hypotension, hypertension, bradycardia, and tachycardia to cardiac arrest.

## Drugs and Decontamination

Give an antidote when there is reasonable certainty of a specific diagnosis. The indications and dosages are discussed subsequently. Decontamination includes skin, eyes, and gastrointestinal decontamination and facilitation for increased drug removal.

### *Decontamination of Skin*

Decontamination means separation of patient from the contaminant, i.e., poison. Many toxins such as OPs and OCLs are readily absorbed through the skin; therefore, systemic absorption can be prevented only by rapid action. The affected areas should be washed with copious amounts of lukewarm water or saline. Area behind the ears, under the nails, and the skinfolds should be carefully washed. For oily substances (pesticides), the skin should be washed at least twice with plain soap and shampoo the hair. Specific decontaminating solutions or solvents (alcohol) are rarely indicated; in some cases, may paradoxically enhance absorption.

### *Gastrointestinal Decontamination*[9,10]

Removal of ingested poisons was a routine part of emergency treatment for decades. Prospective clinical trials have failed to show improved outcomes after gastric emptying. For small and moderate ingestion of most substances, oral activated charcoal alone without prior gastric emptying is recommended. Exceptions are large ingestions of anticholinergic compounds and salicylates, which often delay gastric emptying, and ingestion of sustained release or enteric coated tablets, which may remain intact for several hours.

Gastric emptying is not recommended for ingestion of corrosive agents or petroleum distillates, further esophageal injury or pulmonary aspiration may result. It is also contraindicated in stuporous or comatose patients with absent gag reflexes unless their airway is secured beforehand.

### *Increased Drug Removal*

#### *Urinary Manipulation*

It is useful for drug elimination where the drug undergoes extensive tubular reabsorption and that renal excretion can become a major route of excretion under conditions of forced diuresis. Forced diuresis is hazardous; the risk of complications (pulmonary edema, electrolyte imbalance) outweighs its benefits, and is usually not recommended. It is commonly used for toxicity of acidic drugs (e.g., salicylates, phenobarbital) as they are more rapidly excreted with alkaline urine. Urinary alkalinization is usually achieved by administration of intravenous (IV) sodium bicarbonate (1–2 mEq/kg every 3–4 hours); this may be administered as two 50 mL ampules of 8.4% sodium bicarbonate (each containing 50 mEq of $NaHCO_3$) per liter of 5% dextrose in water infused at 250 mL/hour with aim to keep urinary pH above 7.[11]

#### *Hemodialysis*

The indications for hemodialysis are as follows:

- Known or suspected potentially lethal amounts of dialyzable drug (Table 1)
- Presence of deep coma, apnea, severe hypotension, fluid and electrolyte or acid-base disturbance, or extreme body temperature changes that cannot be corrected by conventional measures
- Poisoning in patients with severe kidney, cardiac, pulmonary, or hepatic disease who will not be able to eliminate toxin by the usual mechanisms.

Continuous renal replacement therapy is of uncertain benefit for elimination of most poisons, but has been used successfully in management of lithium poisoning.[12]

| Table 1: Drugs which can be Removed by Hemodialysis | |
| --- | --- |
| **Poisons** | **Indications** |
| Carbamazepine | Seizures, severe cardiotoxicity; serum levels >60 mg/L |
| Ethylene glycol | Acidosis, serum level >50 mg/dL |
| Lithium | Severe symptoms; level >4 mEq/L more than 12 hours after last dose |
| Methanol | Acidosis, serum levels >50 mg/dL |
| Phenobarbital | Intractable hypotension, acidosis despite maximal supportive care |
| Salicylate | Severe acidosis, central nervous system symptoms, level >100 mg/dL (acute overdose) or >60 mg/dL (chronic intoxication) |
| Theophylline | Serum level >90–100 mg/L (acute) or seizures and serum level >60 mg/L (chronic) |
| Valproic acid | Serum level >900–100 mg/L or deep coma, severe acidosis |

*Repeat Dose Charcoal*

Repeated doses of activated charcoal, 20–30 g orally or via gastric tube every 3–4 hours, may hasten elimination of some drugs (phenytoin, carbamazepine, dapsone) by absorbing drugs excreted into the gut lumen (gut dialysis). Clinical studies have failed to prove better outcome using multiple dose charcoal.[12]

## DIAGNOSIS OF POISONING

Because of its protean manifestations, poisoning and drug overdose should be considered in differential diagnosis of all patients in an acute care setting. The identity of the ingested substance or substances is usually unknown. History is the single most important indicator of toxic ingestion, but occasionally a comatose patient is found or the patient is unable or unwilling to give a coherent history. By performing a directed physical examination and ordering common clinical laboratory tests, the clinician can often make a tentative diagnosis that allows for management of the patient.

## SYMPTOMATIC PATIENT

In symptomatic patients, treatment of life-threatening complications takes precedence over in depth diagnostic evaluation. Every effort should be made to keep the patient alive. Patients with mild symptoms may deteriorate rapidly, which is why all potentially significant exposures should be observed in acute care facility. The following complications may occur, depending upon the type of poisoning.

## Coma

Coma is commonly associated with ingestion of large number of drugs and toxins. The most common cause of death in a comatose patient is respiratory failure, which may occur abruptly. Pulmonary aspiration of gastric contents may also occur, especially in victims who are obtunded or having seizures. Thus, protection of airway and assisted ventilation are the most important treatment measures for any poisoned patient in coma.

Initial emergency management of coma is on lines of airway, breathing, and circulation (ABC). Immediately after stabilizing the coma patient, a "coma cocktail" of thiamine, dextrose, and naloxone should be administered. All comatose or convulsing patients should receive 50–100 mL of 50% dextrose. In alcoholic or severely malnourished patients, 100 mg of thiamine IV over 2–3 minutes should be administered prior to glucose. Naloxone 0.4–2 mg IV may reverse opioid-induced respiratory depression and coma. It is often given empirically in all coma patients. If, however, opioid poisoning is strongly suspected, additional dose of 5–10 mg may be required to reverse the effects. Flumazenil 0.2–0.5 mg IV repeated every 30 seconds or as needed up to a maximum of 3 mg may reverse benzodiazepine-induced coma.

## Agitated or Convulsing Patient

Agitated, violent, or acutely psychotic patients unresponsive to verbal feedback and reduction in environmental stimuli require pharmacological treatment or physical restraints to establish patient safety. Organic causes of agitation other than drug overdose should be considered like drug withdrawal, head trauma with subdural hematoma, intracerebral hemorrhage, hypoglycemia, etc.

Seizures are a major cause of drug-related morbidity and mortality. They are caused by multiple drugs and toxins. Prolonged or repeated seizures may lead to hypoxia, metabolic acidosis, hyperthermia, and rhabdomyolysis, hence require early active intervention.

In an agitated patient, haloperidol (1–5 mg) may be repeated every 30–60 minutes to a total dosage not exceeding 100 mg. Haloperidol lowers seizure threshold and is associated with tardive dyskinesia. For seizures, administer lorazepam, 2–3 mg, or diazepam, 5–10 mg, IV over 2–3 minutes. If seizures are not controlled, consider phenobarbitone, 15–20 mg/kg slowly over no less than 30 minutes; or phenytoin 15 mg/kg IV not exceeding 50 mg/minute. For drug-induced seizures, phenobarbitone is generally preferred over phenytoin. Propofol infusion has also been reported effective for some resistant, drug-induced seizures. Seizures due to a few drugs and toxins may require specific antidotes (Table 2).

| Table 2: Common Compounds Causing Seizures | |
| --- | --- |
| • Amphetamine | • Ethylene glycol |
| • Antihistamines | • Cyclic antidepressants |
| • Antipsychotics | • Isoniazid |
| • Carbamates | • Salicylates |
| • Organochlorines | • Withdrawal from alcohol or sedative-hypnotics |
| • Carbon monoxide | • Organophosphates |
| • Cocaine | |

## Temperature Alteration

Many drugs and toxins have the potential to alter body temperature through a number of different mechanisms. Both hypothermia and hyperthermia are common with intoxication. Hypothermia is caused by peripheral vasodilatation, inhibition of shivering, depression of metabolic activity, and loss of consciousness in cold environment. Hyperthermia occurs due to excessive generation of heat from sustained seizures, muscle rigidity, or an increased metabolic rate as in cocaine intoxication or due to impaired dispersion of heat secondary to decreased sweating as in anticholinergic ingestion. Hyperthermia can also occur due to central cause that alters hypothalamic activity.

Significantly abnormal temperature must be immediately identified and aggressively treated to prevent life-threatening complications. For hypothermic patient, gradual rewarming is preferred unless the patient is in cardiac arrest. Hyperthermia should be aggressively managed by removing all clothes, spraying the patient with tepid water, and fanning the patient. If this is not rapidly effective, or if there is significant muscle rigidity or hyperactivity, induce neuromuscular paralysis with a nondepolarizing neuromuscular blocker (rocuronium, vecuronium). Once paralyzed, the patient must be intubated and mechanically ventilated. Dantrolene (2–5 mg/kg IV) may be effective for hyperthermia associated with muscle rigidity that does not respond to neuromuscular blockade (i.e., malignant hyperthermia).

## Circulatory Manifestations

Circulatory manifestations of drug overdose are common and varied, including cardiac arrest, atrial and ventricular arrhythmias, and hypo- and hypertension.

Hypertension should be treated if the patient is symptomatic or if diastolic blood pressure (BP) is greater than 105–110 mmHg, especially if there is no prior history of hypertension. Hypertensive patient who is agitated or anxious may benefit from a sedative such as lorazepam 2–3 mg IV. For persistent hypertension, administer phentolamine 2–5 mg IV or nitroprusside sodium 0.25–8 µg/kg/minute IV.

For hypotension, most patients respond to empiric treatment with repeated 200 mL IV boluses of 0.9% saline or other isotonic crystalloid up to a total of 1–2 L. If fluid therapy is not successful, dopamine at a dose of 5–15 µg/kg/minute by IV infusion may be given. Pulmonary artery catheterization may be done if hypotension persists. Hypotension due to certain drugs may need specific treatment as in tricyclic antidepressant poisoning sodium bicarbonate (50–100 mEq by IV bolus injection) reverses hypotension; norepinephrine (4–8 µg/minute) is more effective than dopamine. For β-blockers, glucagon 5–10 mg IV may be of value. For calcium channel blocker overdose, calcium chloride at a dose of 1–2 g IV (repeated doses may be necessary) may be administered. Intralipid 20% lipid emulsion has been reported to improve hemodynamics in human case reports; animal studies of intoxication by highly lipid soluble drugs such as bupivacaine, verapamil, bupropion, and clomipramine.[13]

Arrhythmias are often caused by hypoxia or electrolyte imbalance. If ventricular arrhythmias persist, administer lidocaine or amiodarone at usual antiarrhythmic doses. Class 1a agents should be avoided as they may worsen tricyclic antidepressant intoxication.

## Pupil Size

Pupil size can be of help in diagnosis of intoxications as listed in table 3.

## Laboratory Evaluation

Clinical laboratory data includes assessment of three gaps of toxicology: the anion gap, the osmolal gap, and the arterial oxygen saturation gap.

### Oxygen Saturation Gap

Toxins associated with an elevated arterial oxygen gap (>5% difference between calculated from arterial blood gas determination and saturation measured by

**Table 3: Drugs Causing Pupillary Alterations**

| Miosis | Mydriasis | Nystagmus |
|---|---|---|
| • Narcotics | • Deep coma | • Barbiturate |
| • Phenothiazine | • Alcohol | • Phenytoin |
| • Barbiturate | • Atropine | • Phencyclidine |
| • Organophosphate | • Anticholinergics | • Alcohol |
| | • Glutethimide | |
| | • Diphenhydramine | |
| | • Cocaine | |

co-oximetry) include carbon monoxide (CO) and methemoglobin. These toxins interfere with oxygen binding to hemoglobin (Hb) and thereby significantly decrease oxygen content without lowering arterial oxygen tension ($PaO_2$). Oxygen saturation measured by pulse oximetry is falsely high in the setting of these toxins.

### Toxicology Screening

Toxicology screening provides direct evidence of ingestion, but it rarely impacts initial management. Initial supportive measures should never await results of such analysis. If toxicology screen is required, urine is the best specimen (Table 4). Quantitative blood analysis of suspected drugs can be useful for diagnostic and therapeutic reasons, particularly in overdoses involving alcohols, acetaminophen, salicylates, and cyclic antidepressants.

## TREATMENT

After general supportive measures enumerated above, certain drugs or toxins can be managed by specific antidotes. Table 5 lists antidotes for various drugs or toxins.

## Specific Intoxications

### Acetaminophen

Acetaminophen is the most popular over-the-counter analgesic. It is the commonest poisoning in the Western world, especially in the UK. It is uncommon in Indian subcontinent and the developing world. The toxic dose is greater than 150–200 mg/kg or 8–10 g in an average adult. Acetaminophen is primarily metabolized by liver through sulfation (20–46%) and glucuronidation (40–67%). A small percentage is oxidized to a toxic metabolite, N-acetyl-p-benzoquinone imine (NAPQI), by cytochrome P-450, which is quickly detoxified by hepatic

| Table 4: Drugs Detected in Urine | |
| --- | --- |
| **Drugs detected within 30 minutes** | **Drugs detected within 2–3 hours** |
| • Amphetamines | • Acetaminophen |
| • Barbiturates | • Cannabinoids |
| • Benzodiazepines | • Phenothiazine |
| • Cocaine | • Morphine |
| • Opioids | • Propranolol |
| • Phencyclidine | • Ephedrine |

**Table 5: Antidotes to Various Drugs and Poisons**

| Drug/poison | Antidote |
| --- | --- |
| Acetaminophen | N-acetylcysteine |
| Anticholinergics | Physostigmine |
| Anticholinesterases | Atropine |
| Benzodiazepines | Flumazenil |
| Beta-blockers | Glucagon |
| Calcium channel blocker | Calcium chloride, glucagon |
| Cyanide | Amyl nitrite, sodium nitrite, sodium thiosulfate |
| Digoxin | Digoxin-specific antibodies |
| Ethylene glycol | Ethanol |
| Heavy metals | Dimercaprol (BAL), EDTA, penicillamine |
| Opioids | Naloxone |
| Hypoglycemic agents | Dextrose, glucagon |

EDTA, ethylenediaminetetraacetic acid.

stores of glutathione to a nontoxic acetaminophen-mercaptate compound that can be eliminated through renal excretion. However, during toxic overdose a larger proportion is metabolized by cytochrome P-450 to NAPQI, depleting glutathione.

## Clinical Features

The evolution of acetaminophen toxicity is divided into four phases:

*Phase I* refers to the first 24 hours after ingestion. Patients generally remain alert but may experience nausea, vomiting, anorexia, malaise, pallor, or diaphoresis.

*Phase II* occurs 24–72 hours after untreated ingestion. During this period, patient may develop right upper quadrant pain and minor abnormalities of liver function consisting of elevation of hepatic enzymes, prothrombin time and bilirubin.

*Phase III* (72–96 hours after untreated ingestion) is characterized by continued hepatic necrosis, hepatic encephalopathy, disseminated intravascular coagulation, and jaundice. Liver function abnormalities typically peak during phase III. The liver enzymes may rise to 10,000 IU/L or higher. Rare phase III sequel includes hemorrhagic pancreatitis, renal failure and myocardial necrosis.

*Phase IV* occurs 4 days to 2 weeks after ingestion, during which recovery occurs, with return of enzymes to the normal range and without the development of chronic liver damage.

In some patients, there is a rising trend of prothrombin time, ammonia, and bilirubin even though the levels of hepatic enzyme decline indicating fulminant hepatic failure.

## Diagnosis

The diagnosis of acetaminophen toxicity depends on serum levels and time of ingestion. The interpretation of acetaminophen toxicity depends on plotting of Rumack-Matthew nomogram. The nomogram applies to an acetaminophen level measured after 4 hours following and before 24 hours after ingestion.

## Treatment

Charcoal should be given within 1–2 hours of ingestion. One must treat if the serum acetaminophen level is above the nomogram line, i.e., 4-hour level of greater than or equal to 200 µg/mL. If the precise time of ingestion is unknown, a lower threshold of 100 µg/mL at 4 hours may be considered for treatment. Treatment with N-acetylcysteine is most effective if started within 8 hours of ingestion.

The antidote N-acetylcysteine can be given orally or IV. Oral treatment begins with a loading dose of 140 mg/kg followed by 70 mg/kg every 4 hours for 72 hours or 17 doses. The IV regimen includes a loading dose of 150 mg/kg over 1 hour followed by 4-hour infusion of 50 mg/kg, and a 16-hour infusion of 100 mg/kg.[14]

### Amphetamine and Cocaine

Cocaine and amphetamines are widely abused for their euphorigenic and stimulant properties. Both drugs may be smoked, snorted, ingested, or injected. Amphetamines and cocaine produce central nervous system (CNS) stimulation and a generalized increase in central and peripheral sympathetic activity.[15] The toxic dose of each drug is highly variable and depends on the route of administration and individual tolerance. The onset of effects is most rapid after IV route or smoking.[16] Amphetamine derivatives and related drugs include methamphetamine (crystal meth, crank) 3,4-methylenedioxymethamphetamine (MDMA) (ecstasy), ephedrine (herbal ecstasy), and methcathinone (cat).

Toxic effects of cocaine stem from excessive CNS stimulation and inhibition of neuronal uptake of catecholamine. Clinical features include anxiety, tremulousness, tachycardia, hypertension, diaphoresis, dilated pupils, agitation, muscular hyperactivity, and psychosis.[17] Muscle hyperactivity may lead to metabolic acidosis and rhabdomyolysis. In severe intoxication, seizures and hyperthermia may occur. Sustained or severe hypertension may result in intracranial hemorrhage, aortic dissection, or myocardial infarction. Hyponatremia has been reported after

MDMA use. Respiratory complications include status asthmaticus, upper airway obstruction, pulmonary hypertension, barotrauma, pulmonary edema, and alveolar hemorrhage.[16,18]

## Treatment

The diagnosis is supported by finding amphetamines, cocaine, or the cocaine metabolite benzoylecgonine in the urine. Blood screening is generally not sensitive enough to detect these drugs. Emergency treatment includes ABC and rapid lowering of body temperature in patients who have hyperthermia. Treat agitation, psychosis, or seizures with a benzodiazepine such as lorazepam, 2–3 mg IV. Add phenobarbitone 15 mg/kg IV for persistent seizures.

Hypertension should be treated with a vasodilator agent such as phentolamine (1–5 mg IV) or a combined $\alpha$- and $\beta$-blocker such as labetalol (10–20 mg IV). A pure $\beta$-blocker such as propranolol should not be used as it may result in paradoxical worsening of hypertension due to unopposed $\alpha$-adrenergic effect.

Tachycardia or tachyarrhythmias should be treated with a short-acting $\beta$-blocker like esmolol (25–100 µg/kg/minute by IV infusion).

### Aluminum Phosphide Poisoning

Aluminum phosphide is a very common cause of poisoning in northwest and central India.[19] It is available as tablets of 3 g, which contains 56% aluminum phosphide and 44% ammonium carbonate. Toxicity of aluminum phosphide is due to phosphine, which is released when it comes in contact with moisture or hydrochloric acid. The precise cellular mechanism of phosphine is not clear. It is stipulated that it acts by preventing the uptake of oxygen by mitochondria. Clinically a myriad of symptoms are produced by ingestion of aluminum phosphide. Immediately after ingestion, all patients develop nausea, vomiting, retrosternal burning, and in case of significant poisoning, hypotension and shock.[19,20]

Oliguria develops in a few patients. Adult respiratory distress syndrome develops in patients with severe intoxication. Most patients develop myocarditis manifested by variable electrocardiographic changes ranging from bradyarrhythmias to tachyarrhythmias. Other complications include disseminated intravascular coagulation, intravascular hemolysis, congestive cardiac failure, hepatic failure, and rarely pericarditis. Patients generally remain conscious till cerebral anoxia due to shock supervenes, resulting in drowsiness, delirium, and coma.[19]

## Management

The diagnosis is made by history of ingestion. The diagnosis of aluminum phosphide poisoning can be made by detecting phosphine in exhaled air or in stomach contents. There is no specific antidote for this poisoning and the treatment is supportive. Gastric lavage should be done with potassium permanganate within 1 hour of ingestion. For management of hypotension, IV fluids should be given judiciously as central venous pressure is generally high in these patients. If the hypotension does not respond, then dopamine/dobutamine may be used to maintain the systolic BP above 80 mmHg. Magnesium sulfate, a membrane stabilizer which can reverse arrhythmias, has been used. Though arrhythmias improve, mortality does not decline. In severe cases, compromised adrenal function has been reported. Corticosteroids have been used, but the outcome remains poor.[21]

### *Carbon Monoxide Poisoning*

Carbon monoxide poisoning is the third leading cause of unintentional poisoning death in the US.[22] Incidence of CO toxicity in developing countries is not available. Nonfatal incidences are more common than the fatal ones and misdiagnosis is usual.[22] CO poisoning occurs due to exposure to internal combustion engines in poorly ventilated places, fires, smoke inhalation and industrial accidents. Incidence tends to increase during winter months.

### *Pathophysiology*

Carbon monoxide has 220 times more affinity to Hb than oxygen. It binds reversibly to Hb and its dissociation curve runs parallel to oxygen dissociation curve, but moves in opposite direction, i.e., CO curve shifts to right whereas oxygen dissociation curve shifts to left resulting in significant tissue hypoxia.[22] Due to its higher affinity to myoglobin, CO also enhances the risk of myocardial ischemia. Further, CO activates platelets and neutrophils, enhances formation of oxygen free radicals that lead to lipid peroxidation and tissue destruction especially in the neural tissue. It is not surprising that presenting symptoms of CO toxicity are predominantly neurological and cardiovascular.

### *Clinical Features*

Symptoms of toxicity are variable and nonspecific. Careful history of exposure is important. Commonly, patients complain of fatigue, nausea, vomiting, dizziness, and headache. As the severity increases, they develop ataxia, nystagmus, impaired judgments, and become unconscious. They can also develop dysrhythmia, myocardial dysfunction leading to hypotension and metabolic acidosis. Presence of retinal hemorrhages strongly indicates CO poisoning. Patients can also have cyanosis and cherry-red color of the skin. In pregnant patients, there is an increase risk of fetal death. Later on, the patient may develop either persistent or delayed neurologic sequalae.

*Diagnosis*

The diagnosis is confirmed by CO oximetry of the blood which shows elevation of COHb levels beyond 10%. Severe poisoning is usually associated with levels of more than 40%. Pulse oximeter usually gives falsely high values of saturation, hence must not be relied.

*Treatment*

Patient should be moved to a safer environment to prevent additional exposure. The rescuer should ensure self-protection by taking necessary precautions to avoid exposure to toxic fumes before attempting patient's evacuation. If the patient is not unconscious, 100% oxygen using a tight mask with a flow rate of at least 10 L/minute should be given. In case the patient is unconscious, he should be intubated and ventilated with 100% oxygen till COHb level reaches 5%. Wherever facility exists/available, hyperbaric oxygen should be preferred in severely poisoned cases.[22]

## Insecticide Poisoning (Organophosphates, Carbamate, Organochlorine, Herbicide)

There are two major classes of insecticides that are used in commercial agriculture and home gardening, the OPs (malathion, parathion) and the carbamate (carbaryl, aldicarb). Insecticides can be absorbed from mouth, skin, conjunctiva, gastrointestinal tract, and/or respiratory tract. The cause of poisoning varies from suicidal attempt to accidental exposure. Signs and symptoms of acute poisoning generally occur within the first 12–24 hours after exposure.

*Organophosphate Poisoning*

Commonly used OPs include malathion, parathion, chlorpyrifos, dichlorophos, and phorate. OPs act by inhibiting the enzyme cholinesterase leading to accumulation of acetylcholine at neuromuscular junction and nerve terminal resulting in overstimulation of acetylcholine receptors. This initial overstimulation is followed by paralysis of cholinergic transmission in the CNS, autonomic ganglia, parasympathetic and some sympathetic nerve endings, and in some somatic nerves. A cholinergic crisis results in central and peripheral syndrome. OPs bind irreversibly to cholinesterase, thus inactivating the enzyme through the process of phosphorylation. The aging that is permanent binding of the OPs to the enzyme requires 24–48 hours to occur. Once aging occurs, only new enzymatic resynthesis must occur over a period of weeks before the clinical symptoms resolve and normal enzymatic function returns.

*Diagnosis:* In most of the developing countries, diagnosis of OP poisoning is clinical. It can be confirmed by the assays of plasma and red blood cell (RBC) cholinesterases. Plasma cholinesterase assays are more readily available although estimation of RBC cholinesterases is preferred over serum cholinesterases. Serum and RBC cholinesterase are usually depressed at least 50% below baseline in severe intoxication.

*Treatment:* Primarily, treatment of OP poisoning includes decontamination, supportive therapy including mechanical ventilation and definitive therapy in form of antidotes like atropine and oximes.

*Decontamination:* OP compounds are highly lipophilic readily absorbed from skin, gut and lungs. Clothes should be removed and patient should be given a thorough wash with soap and water. Gastric lavage is done routinely but is not of great help. Activated charcoal (single or multiple doses) though found to be effective in animal models of OP poisoning within first hour is not effective in humans.[23] Airway protection should be a routine whenever lavage is done.

*Supportive therapy:* Large proportion of these patients develops respiratory failure secondary to depolarizing muscle paralysis and overwhelming bronchorrhea. Airway must be protected early (preferably rapid sequence) followed by control of breathing and circulation. Oxygenation should be started with an aim to have saturations more than 88%; the threshold for initiation of mechanical ventilation should be low. In case of seizures, preferred treatment is benzodiazepines (lorazepam/diazepam/midazolam in usual doses) along with atropine.[24]

Respiratory muscle weakness may persist and causes difficulty in weaning, in spite of apparent improvement in general condition and resolution of symptoms. Therefore, patients need close observation especially for respiratory and heart rate. Fall in $SpO_2$ or rise in $PaCO_2$ are late signs.

*Specific therapy:* Atropine is the specific antidote in OP poisoning. It is usually given as 2–5 mg IV bolus (0.05 mg/kg IV in children), escalated (double) every 3–5 minutes until bronchial secretions and wheezing stops. Once the patient is fully atropinized, i.e., heart rate is more than 80 and secretions are dry; atropine infusion is set up by giving 20–30% of the total amount that was required to atropinize the patient initially every hour. The infusion dose is maintained for 2–3 days for full atropinization, then the dose is daily reduced by one-fourth to one-third of the previous day's dose.[25] Atropine is associated with anticholinergic side effects including psychosis. The aim of therapy is to have heart rate more than 80, drying of secretions without dilatation of pupils, and gut paralysis (observe abdominal sounds). Glycopyrronium bromide (glycopyrrolate) can be used in place or together with atropine or if CNS side effects of later develop.[24]

## Oximes

Theoretical and experimental basis of the use of oximes in OP poisoning is strong. In humans, especially in case of self-harm, the data for their use is conflicting.[24,26-28] It has been argued that efficacy of oximes depends not only on the amount but also on the nature of consumed compound (dimethyl vs. the diethyl, former being more resistant), dosages, time of their administration, aging, and reactivation kinetics. There is a therapeutic window during which oximes may be effective. The window in turn depends on extent and rate of aging of acetylcholinesterase. Further, the type of oxime used is also a decisive factor in addition to their dosage (obidoxime is 9 times more active than pralidoxime).[27] Oximes have their own side effects. Rapid administration of oxime can cause respiratory arrest in patients having shallow respiration.[28] In the presence of OP compounds, they get converted to stable phosphoryl oximes. This further leads to the restriction of their ability to reactivate phosphorylated cholinesterases and have been blamed for the variable response of oximes in OP toxicity.

In summary, evidence is mixed for the effectiveness and use of oximes in OP poisoning. The World Health Organization guidelines recommend to give high-dose oximes in OP poisoning. As of today, the recommended dosages are: pralidoxime chloride 30 mg/kg bolus followed by 8–10 mg/kg/hour or obidoxime 250 mg bolus followed by 750 mg/24 hours, until at least 12 hours after stopping of atropine.[24]

## Carbamate Poisoning

Carbamates are cholinesterase inhibitors that are structurally related to OPs. Commonly used carbamates are Sevin, Baygon, and Lannate. They transiently and reversibly inhibit cholinesterase enzymes unlike OPs. Regeneration of the enzyme occurs within few hours by dissociation of the carbamyl-cholinesterase complex. Clinical features of carbamate poisoning are similar to OP poisoning but of shorter duration. Carbamates do not readily penetrate the CNS and hence less CNS effects are seen.

*Treatment*: Cholinesterase levels and thus enzymatic activity usually returns to normal within 4–6 hours, therefore, measurement of RBC cholinesterase level is not useful. Initial treatment is similar to OP poisoning. Atropine is the antidote of choice and is administered for muscarinic symptoms as is done for OP poisoning. There is little need for pralidoxime in carbamate poisoning.[29]

## Organochlorine Poisoning

Organochlorine compounds include dichloro-diphenyl-trichloroethane, chlordane, hexachlorocyclohexane, and aldrin. OCLs are well absorbed by ingestion, inhalation, and minimally through skin.

*Mechanism of action*: These agents are CNS stimulants and work by inhibiting gamma-aminobutyric acid (GABA) and glycine pathways. This leads to inhibition of chloride channels preventing influx of Cl⁻ resulting in neuroexcitation, i.e., inhibitory control is lost.[30]

Organochlorines are highly lipid soluble, resulting slow redistribution, prolongation of elimination half-life, and thus increased duration of toxicity. Clinical features include predominance of neurological symptoms ranging from hyperexcitability, irritability, delirium, myoclonus, and facial paresthesias in mild toxicity to seizures and status epilepticus in severe toxicity. In addition, these agents may produce myocardial irritability with ventricular fibrillation.

*Management*: History is important for making the diagnosis. Laboratory evaluation is generally not helpful but these agents can be detected in serum and urine. Treatment includes oxygen administration, intubation to treat hypoxia secondary to seizures, aspiration, and respiratory failure. Seizures are treated with benzodiazepines (lorazepam 0.04 mg/kg, midazolam 0.05 mg/kg or diazepam 0.2 mg/kg). If they still persist, phenobarbitone or anesthesia with sodium thiopental may have to be used. Electroencephalographic monitoring should be a routine in these cases to observe seizure activity.

Atropine and epinephrine should be avoided for the control of dysrhythmia in OCL sensitized myocardium. Cholestyramine, a bile salt-binding substance, has been found to be helpful in reducing the absorption of these compounds (4 g 4 times/day for at least 2–3 days for ingestional poisoning).[31]

## Herbicide Poisoning

Herbicides are pesticides used to kill weeds. Herbicides may be classified as chlorophenoxy, bipyridyl, and urea-substituted compounds. Chlorophenoxy compounds dioxins and furans are the common chemicals in this group. Other agents are 2,4-dichlorophenoxyacetic acid and 4-chloro-2-methylphenoxyacetic acid.

The metabolic pathway and mechanism related to toxicity are unknown. Skeletal muscle toxicity can result in respiratory failure or rhabdomyolysis. Toxicity can result from inhalation or ingestion. Clinical features include eye and mucous membrane irritation. After ingestion, nausea, vomiting, and diarrhea follow. Cardiovascular findings include hypotension, tachycardia, and dysrhythmias. Muscle toxicity manifests by muscle tenderness, fasciculation, and myotonia with resulting rhabdomyolysis.[32]

*Treatment*: Diagnosis is based on history of exposure. There is metabolic acidosis and hepatorenal dysfunction. Myoglobinuria and elevated creatinine levels indicate rhabdomyolysis. Treatment is supportive, including decontamination measures and respiratory support. Alkalinization is not of any proven benefit, but may be tried for severe toxicity.[33]

## Bipyridyl Compounds

Paraquat and diquat are nonselective herbicides included in this class. Ingestion is responsible for maximum of paraquat-related deaths. Paraquat is distributed to most organs with maximum concentration in lungs and kidneys. Acute exposure causes liver and renal necrosis that is followed after weeks by pulmonary fibrosis. Paraquat accumulates in the alveolar cells of the lungs where it is transformed to reactive oxygen species, the superoxide anion. This anion is responsible for lipid peroxidation causing degradation of the membranes. Paraquat and oxygen enhance each other's toxicity by sustaining the redox cycle. Myocardial injury and necrosis of adrenal gland may occur. Paraquat's caustic effects cause local skin irritation and ulceration of the mucous membranes. Hypovolemia occurs due to gastrointestinal losses and decreased oral intake. Cardiovascular collapse may occur early in severe toxicity. Multisystem effects follow including gastrointestinal corrosion, acute tubular necrosis, and extensive pulmonary injury. Seizures, gastrointestinal perforation, hemorrhage, and hepatic failure may occur. Pulmonary fibrosis leading to refractory hypoxemia occurs 5 days to several weeks later. Metabolic (lactic) acidosis is common as a result of pulmonary effects (hypoxemia) and multisystem failure.[34]

*Treatment*: Early diagnosis and treatment are essential. Diagnosis is based on history. Qualitative and quantitative analyses for paraquat in serum and urine can help in diagnosis. A 10-hour level of greater than 0.4 mg/L carries a high probability of death.[35,36] The goal of early and vigorous decontamination is to prevent pulmonary toxicity. Early treatment is supportive. An attempt should be made to prevent superoxide radical formation by using low inspired oxygen to produce therapeutic hypoxemia with the goal of reducing pulmonary toxicity. The use of low oxygen mixtures [fraction of inspired oxygen ($FiO_2$) <21%] with positive pressure ventilation reduces pulmonary toxicity. It is suggested that a higher $FiO_2$ may only be used when arterial oxygen pressure is less than 40 mmHg.[32] Maintaining intravascular volumes and urine output are important to prevent prerenal failure. Immediate gut contamination with activated charcoal must be done.

Immunosuppressive therapy (cyclophosphamide with dexamethasone) has shown possible benefit in anecdotal reports.[37] In a retrospective analysis of 89 patients, 5 patients with severe paraquat poisoning were treated with IV methyl-prednisolone (15/mg/kg body weight) for 3 days and IV cyclophosphamide (10 mg/kg body weight) for 2 consecutive days followed by IV dexamethasone

4 mg thrice daily until recovery or death. Two of the five patients survived. In a meta-analysis comprising of 12 studies, the use of immunosuppressive therapy was associated with successful treatment of one out of four treated patients.[38]

## Opioids

The term opioid is an all-inclusive term for antagonists, endogenous, and exogenous substances that possess morphine-like activity. The most commonly abused opioids are heroin and methadone. Prescription and illicit opioids (morphine, codeine, oxycodone, fentanyl, and others) are popular drugs of abuse and the cause of frequent hospitalizations for overdose.[39] These drugs have widely varying potencies and durations of action; some of the illicit fentanyl derivatives are up to 2,000 times more potent than morphine. All of these agents decrease CNS activity and sympathetic outflow by acting on opiate receptors in the brain.

Mild intoxication is characterized by euphoria, drowsiness, and constricted pupils. More severe intoxication may cause hypotension, bradycardia, hypothermia, coma, and respiratory arrest. Pulmonary edema may occur.[40] Death is usually due to apnea or pulmonary aspiration of gastric contents. Propoxyphene may cause seizure and prolongation of QRS interval.[41] Methadone has been associated with QT interval prolongation and torsades de pointes. With meperidine, the metabolite normeperidine probably causes seizures and is most likely to accumulate after repeat dosing in patients with chronic kidney disease.[42]

*Treatment*: Naloxone is a specific opioid antagonist that can rapidly reverse the signs of narcotic intoxication. Although it is structurally related to opioids, it has no agonist effects of its own. It is given at a dose of 0.4–2 mg IV, a repeat dose may be given to awaken the patient. Very large doses (10–20 mg) may be required for patients intoxicated by some opioids (propoxyphene, codeine, fentanyl derivatives). The duration of effect of naloxone is only 2–3 hours; repeated doses may be necessary for patients intoxicated by long-acting drugs such as methadone. Continuous observation for at least 3 hours after the last dose of naloxone is mandatory.[43] In severest forms associated with respiratory depression, intubation and ventilation may be required.

## CONCLUSION

Accidental or self-inflicted poisoning is an important preventable cause of morbidity and mortality. It is medical emergency and requires a high index of clinical suspicion. Treatment involves stabilization and instituting a specific antidote in order to prevent further organ damage and/or death.

> ## Editor's Comment
>
> *Acute poisoning is an important and challenging field where a good knowledge of toxicology and critical care is needed to best manage the patient. It is a frequently encountered emergency in the casualty. One needs to be able to diagnose the clinical feature of a particular type of poisoning as the history at times may not be forthcoming. Methods to limit the absorption of the poison and its specific antidote need to be known. Also, steps to maintain hemodynamic stability and breathing need to be initiated. In the developing world, organophosphate compounds and aluminum phosphide are the common cause of poisoning. The diagnosis of these poisoning is based on clinical grounds and one needs to be familiar with their signs and symptoms. For organophosphate poisoning, a specific antidote exists; but for aluminum phosphide, there is no specific antidote and the management is largely supportive. The treatment of poisoning will vary depending upon the poison, its route of entry, and the drugs effect on different organs in the body. The supportive care in terms of maintaining hemodynamic stability, supporting breathing, and other organ function remains largely the same.*
>
> ***Randeep Guleria***

## REFERENCES


1. Litovitz TL, Smilkstein M, Felberg L, Klein-Schwartz W, Berlin R, Morgan JL. 1996 annual report of the American Association of Poison Control Centers Toxic Exposure Surveillance System. *Am J Emerg Med.* 1997;15(5):447-500.
2. Spiller HA, Winter ML, Mann KV, Borys DJ, Muir S, Krenzelok EP. Five-year multicenter retrospective review of cyclobenzaprine toxicity. *J Emerg Med.* 1995;13(6):781-5.
3. Singh S, Sharma BK, Wahi PL, Anand BS, Chugh KS. Spectrum of acute poisoning in adults (10 year experience). *J Assoc Physicians India.* 1984;32(7):561-3.
4. Gunnell D, Eddleston M, Phillips MR, Konradsen F. The global distribution of fatal pesticide self-poisoning: systematic review. *BMC Public Health.* 2007;7:357.
5. Thomas M, Anandan S, Kuruvilla PJ, Singh PR, David S. Profile of hospital admissions following acute poisoning—experiences from a major teaching hospital in south India. *Adverse Drug React Toxicol Rev.* 2000;19(4):313-7.
6. Srivastava A, Peshin SS, Kaleekal T, Gupta SK. An epidemiological study of poisoning cases reported to the National Poisons Information Centre, All India Institute of Medical Sciences, New Delhi. *Hum Exp Toxicol.* 2005;24(6):279-85.
7. Agarwal SB. A clinical, biochemical, neurobehavioral, and sociopsychological study of 190 patients admitted to hospital as a result of acute organophosphorus poisoning. *Environ Res.* 1993;62(1):63-70.
8. Singh D, Jit I, Tyagi S. Changing trends in acute poisoning in Chandigarh zone: a 25-year autopsy experience from a tertiary care hospital in northern India. *Am J Forensic Med Pathol.* 1999;20(2):203-10.
9. Rudolph JP. Automated gastric lavage and a comparison of 0.9% normal saline solution and tap water irrigant. *Ann Emerg Med.* 1985;14(12):1156-9.
10. Winchester JF. Active methods of detoxification. In: Haddad LM, Winchester JF (Eds). Clinical Management of Poisoning and Drug Overdose, 2nd edition. Philadelphia: WB Saunders; 1990.

11. Ismail N, Becker BN. Principles of and techniques for dialysis, plasmapheresis, and hemoperfusion: Common poisoning and drug overdose. In: Jacobson H, Striker GE, Klahr S (Eds). The Principles and Practice of Nephrology, 2nd edition. St. Louis: Mosby; 1988.

12. Brahmi N, Kouraichi N, Thabet H, Amamou M. Influence of activated charcoal on the pharmacokinetics and the clinical features of carbamazepine poisoning. *Am J Emerg Med*. 2006;24(4):440-3.

13. Sirianni AJ, Osterhoudt KC, Calello DP, Muller AA, Waterhouse MR, Goodkin MB, et al. Use of lipid emulsion in the resuscitation of a patient with prolonged cardiovascular collapse after overdose of bupropion and lamotrigine. *Ann Emerg Med*. 2008;51(4):412-5, 415.e1.

14. Temple AR, Mrazik TJ. More on extended-release acetaminophen. *N Engl J Med*. 1995;333(22):1508-9.

15 Beckman KJ, Parker RB, Hariman RJ, Gallastegui JL, Javaid JI, Bauman JL. Hemodynamic and electrophysiological actions of cocaine. Effects of sodium bicarbonate as an antidote in dogs. *Circulation*. 1991;83(5):1799-807.

16. Tashkin DP, Kleerup EC, Koyal SN, Marques JA, Goldman MD. Acute effects of inhaled and i.v. cocaine on airway dynamics. *Chest*. 1996;110(4):904-10.

17. Mathias S, Lubman DI, Hides L. Substance-induced psychosis: a diagnostic conundrum. *J Clin Psychiatry*. 2008;69(3):358-67.

18. Osborn HH, Tang M, Bradley K, Duncan BR. New-onset bronchospasm or recrudescence of asthma associated with cocaine abuse. *Acad Emerg Med*. 1997;4(7):689-92.

19. Chugh SN, Chugh K, Ram S, Malhotra KC. Electrocardiographic abnormalities in aluminium phosphide poisoning with special reference to its incidence, pathogenesis, mortality and histopathology. *J Indian Med Assoc*. 1991;89(2):32-5.

20. Bajaj R, Wasir HS, Aggarwal R. Aluminium phosphide poisoning. Clinical toxicity and outcome in eleven intensively monitored patients. *Nat Med J India*. 1988;1:270-4.

21. Chugh SN, Ram S, Sharma A, Arora BB, Saini AS, Malhotra KC. Adrenocortical involvement in aluminium phosphide poisoning. *Indian J Med Res*. 1989;90:289-94.

22. Wolf SJ, Lavonas EJ, Sloan EP, Jagoda AS; American College of Emergency Physicians. Clinical policy: critical issues in the management of adult patients presenting to the emergency department with acute carbon monoxide poisoning. *Ann Emerg Med*. 2008;51(2):138-52.

23. Eddleston M, Juszczak E, Buckley NA, Senarathna L, Mohamed F, Dissanayake W, et al. Multiple-dose activated charcoal in acute self-poisoning: a randomised controlled trial. *Lancet*. 2008;371(9612):579-87.

24. Eddleston M, Buckley NA, Eyer P, Dawson AH. Management of acute organophosphorus pesticide poisoning. *Lancet*. 2008;371(9612):597-607.

25. Bhattarai MD, Singh DL, Chalise BS, Koirala P. A case report and overview of organophosphate (OP) poisoning. *Kathmandu Univ Med J (KUMJ)*. 2006;4(1):100-4.

26. Johnson S, Peter JV, Thomas K, Jeyaseelan L, Cherian AM. Evaluation of two treatment regimens of pralidoxime (1 gm single bolus dose vs. 12 gm infusion) in the management of organophosphorus poisoning. *J Assoc Physicians India*. 1996;44(8):529-31.

27. Pawar KS, Bhoite RR, Pillay CP, Chavan SC, Malshikare DS, Garad SG. Continuous pralidoxime infusion versus repeated bolus injection to treat organophosphorus pesticide poisoning: a randomised controlled trial. *Lancet*. 2006;368(9553):2136-41.

28. Eddleston M, Eyer P, Worek F, Juszczak E, Alder N, Mohamed F, et al. Pralidoxime in acute organophosphorus insecticide poisoning—a randomised controlled trial. *PLoS Med*. 2009;6(6):e1000104.

29. Xue SZ, Ding XJ, Ding Y. Clinical observation and comparison of the effectiveness of several oxime cholinesterase reactivators. *Scand J Work Environ Health*. 1985;11 Suppl 4:46-8.

30. Roberts DM, Dissanayake W, Rezvi Sheriff MH, Eddleston M. Refractory status epilepticus following self-poisoning with the organochlorine pesticide endosulfan. *J Clin Neurosci*. 2004;11(7):760-2.

31. Vale C, Fonfria E, Bujons J, Messeguer A, Rodríguez-Farré E, Suñol C. The organochlorine pesticides gamma-hexachlorocyclohexane (lindane), α-endosulfan and dieldrin differentially interact with GABA(A) and glycine-gated chloride channels in primary cultures of cerebellar granule cells. *Neuroscience*. 2003;117(2):397-403.

32. Cohn WJ, Boylan JJ, Blanke RV, Fariss MW, Howell JR, Guzelian PS. Treatment of chlordecone (Kepone) toxicity with cholestyramine. Results of a controlled clinical trial. *N Engl J Med.* 1978;298(5):243-8.

33. Suskind RR, Hertzberg VS. Human health effects of 2,4,5-T and its toxic contaminants. *JAMA.* 1984;251(18):2372-80.

34. Vale JA, Meredith TJ, Buckley BM. Paraquat poisoning: clinical features and immediate general management. *Hum Toxicol.* 1987;6(1):41-7.

35. Bismuth C, Baud FJ, Garnier R, Muszinski J, Houze P. Paraquat poisoning: biological presentation. *J Toxicol Clin Exp.* 1988;8(3):211-8.

36. Hart TB, Nevitt A, Whitehead A. A new statistical approach to the prognostic significance of plasma paraquat concentrations. *Lancet.* 1984;2(8413):1222-3.

37. Lin JL, Lin-Tan DT, Chen KH, Huang WH. Repeated pulse of methylprednisolone and cyclophosphamide with continuous dexamethasone therapy for patients with severe paraquat poisoning. *Crit Care Med.* 2006;34(2):368-73.

38. Agarwal R, Srinivas R, Aggarwal AN, Gupta D. Immunosuppressive therapy in lung injury due to paraquat poisoning: a meta-analysis. *Singapore Med J.* 2007;48(11):1000-5.

39. Shadnia S, Soltaninejad K, Heydari K, Sasanian G, Abdollahi M. Tramadol intoxication: a review of 114 cases. *Hum Exp Toxicol.* 2008;27(3):201-5.

40. Sternbach G. William Osler: narcotic-induced pulmonary edema. *J Emerg Med.* 1983;1(2):165-7.

41. Ng B, Alvear M. Dextropropoxyphene addiction—a drug of primary abuse. *Am J Drug Alcohol Abuse.* 1993;19(2):153-8.

42. Hershey LA. Meperidine and central neurotoxicity. *Ann Intern Med.* 1983;98(4):548-9.

43. Piper TM, Stancliff S, Rudenstine S, Sherman S, Nandi V, Clear A, et al. Evaluation of a naloxone distribution and administration program in New York City. *Subst Use Misuse.* 2008;43(7):858-70.

World Clin Pulm Crit Care Med. 2016;4(1):123-36.

# Chronic Respiratory Failure

[1]John P Willoughby MD BS, [1]Nicholas Raush MD, [2],*Jennifer Trevor MD

[1]Department of Internal Medicine, University of Alabama at Birmingham
Birmingham, Alabama, United States
[2]Department of Pulmonary, Allergy, and Critical Care Medicine
University of Alabama at Birmingham, Birmingham, Alabama, United States

## ABSTRACT

Chronic respiratory failure is manifested by hypercapnia or hypoxemia, which develops as a result of different etiologies and requires different methods of management. Hypoxemia is caused by a low inspired oxygen fraction, low barometric pressure, alveolar hypoventilation, diffusion impairment, ventilation/perfusion mismatch, or right-to-left shunt. Carbon dioxide removal is dependent on the mechanical process of ventilation, and hypercapnia is the result of dysfunction of the airways, nervous system, chest wall, or diaphragm. The mainstays of therapy for chronic respiratory failure include supplemental oxygen and positive pressure ventilation. Long-term oxygen therapy is the standard of care for chronic hypoxemia and likely improves survival and quality of life for most patients. Positive pressure ventilation is subdivided into noninvasive ventilation, in which positive pressure is applied via masks or nose/mouth pieces, and invasive ventilation, which requires endotracheal intubation and necessitates tracheostomy when long-term ventilation is required. Patients with sufficiently stable disease and a good long-term prognosis may be candidates for home invasive ventilation.

## INTRODUCTION

The primary function of the lungs is to facilitate the uptake of oxygen into the blood and to remove carbon dioxide ($CO_2$). When the lungs are unable to perform this function, the term *respiratory failure* is used. Respiratory failure can be further subdivided into hypoxemic (type I) or hypercapnic (type II) (Table 1).

---

*Corresponding author
*Email:* jtrevor@uab.edu

## Table 1: Chronic Respiratory Failure

| Type I (Hypoxemic) | Type II (Hypercapnic) |
|---|---|
| • Alveolar hypoventilation | • Central nervous system |
| • Diffusion impairment | • Chest wall |
| • V/Q mismatch | • Neuromuscular |
| • Right-to-left shunt | • Pulmonary |

## Table 2: Causes of Chronic Hypoxemic Respiratory Failure

| | |
|---|---|
| Alveolar hypoventilation | Chronic obstructive pulmonary disease, obstructive sleep apnea, obesity hypoventilation syndrome, critical illness myopathy, central nervous system trauma |
| Diffusion impairment | Interstitial lung disease, pulmonary edema |
| V/Q mismatch | Chronic pulmonary thromboembolism, emphysema |
| Right-to-left shunt | Liver failure, intracardiac shunts, chronic pulmonary thromboembolism |

## Table 3: Causes of Chronic Hypercapnic Respiratory Failure

| | |
|---|---|
| Central nervous system (CNS) | CNS trauma, central sleep apnea, coma |
| Chest wall | Chest wall trauma, kyphoscoliosis/spinal deformities, diaphragm pathology, obesity |
| Neuromuscular | Poliomyelitis, critical illness myopathy, Guillain-Barré syndrome, spine trauma, muscular dystrophy |
| Pulmonary | Chronic obstructive pulmonary disease, asthma, airway obstruction, obstructive sleep apnea |

Hypoxemic respiratory failure is defined as having a partial pressure of arterial oxygen ($PaO_2$) of less than 60 mmHg with a low or normal partial pressure of carbon dioxide ($PCO_2$). Hypercapnic respiratory failure is defined as a $PCO_2$ of greater than 50 mmHg with a normal or low $PaO_2$. These two categories can be further divided into acute or chronic variants. Chronic hypercapnic respiratory failure is differentiated from acute failure based on having a normal pH due to compensated serum bicarbonate levels. Chronic hypoxemic respiratory failure differs from acute hypoxemic respiratory failure in the time to onset of the disorder and change from baseline.[1,2] Hypoxemic respiratory failure (Table 2) and hypercapnic respiratory failure (Table 3) differ in their etiologies and management. In addition to treating the underlying cause, hypoxemic failure is managed with supplementary oxygen, while hypercapnic failure is managed with interventions that improve ventilation.

# CHRONIC HYPOXEMIC RESPIRATORY FAILURE

## Physiology

Oxygen enters the body through the oropharynx and moves through the airway to the alveoli through the process of ventilation. This process is regulated by the central nervous system (CNS), chest wall, diaphragm, and elastic properties of the lung. Dysfunction of any of these systems can interrupt the process of oxygenation.[3] Once oxygen is in the alveolar space, its entry into the blood is determined by the diffusion gradient of oxygen across the alveolar-capillary membrane, the properties of the membrane itself, and the rate at which blood flows through the capillary bed. The diffusion gradient is determined by the difference in the partial pressure of oxygen between the alveoli and the capillary blood. In a healthy lung, oxygen diffuses very rapidly across this barrier making oxygenation of the blood dependent on the rate at which the capillaries are perfused.[4]

Once an oxygen molecule reaches the circulation, it binds to hemoglobin (Hb) or dissolves within the plasma. The arterial oxygen content ($CaO_2$) can be described numerically as follows:

$$CaO_2 = (1.34 \times Hb \times SaO_2) + (0.003 \times PaO_2)$$

In the above equation, $SaO_2$ is the oxygen saturation of Hb, and $PaO_2$ is the dissolved oxygen in plasma. The $SaO_2$ is measured with pulse oximetry, and the $PaO_2$ can be measured by arterial blood gas (ABG) analysis.

## Pathophysiology

There are six commonly cited etiologies for hypoxemic respiratory failure: (i) low inspired oxygen fraction, (ii) low barometric pressure, (iii) alveolar hypoventilation, (iv) diffusion impairment, (v) ventilation/perfusion (V/Q) mismatch, and (vi) right-to-left shunt. Low inspired oxygen fraction refers to situations where the lungs are ventilated with air with a decreased percentage of oxygen, such as in the administration of oxygen-poor gas. Low barometric pressure occurs in situations where the percentage of oxygen may be normal but less oxygen is carried due to low pressure, such as at high altitudes. These two etiologies are more common in acute settings and as such will not be discussed further.

### Alveolar Hypoventilation

Alveolar hypoventilation, as an etiology of chronic hypoxemic respiratory failure, encompasses disorders that are caused by chronically decreased ventilation. These causes overlap with those that cause chronic hypercapnic respiratory failure. The alveolar gas equation is as follows:

$$PAO_2 = PiO_2 - (PACO_2/RQ)$$

From the above equation, we can infer that conditions which chronically increase the alveolar carbon dioxide content ($PACO_2$) will cause a concurrent decrease in the alveolar oxygen content ($PAO_2$). This will in turn decrease diffusion of oxygen into the bloodstream. Therefore, conditions resulting in a severe increase in $PACO_2$ can cause combined hypoxemic and hypercapnic respiratory failure. These conditions include chronic obstructive pulmonary disease (COPD), obstructive sleep apnea (OSA), and obesity hypoventilation syndrome (OHS), among others. We can also derive from the above equation that increasing the total amount of inspired oxygen ($PiO_2$) will overcome the hypoxemic portion of the respiratory failure.

## *Diffusion Impairment*

Diffusion impairment refers to conditions that effect the diffusion of oxygen from the alveoli into the bloodstream. While $CO_2$ diffuses rapidly across this barrier, oxygen transport can be profoundly interrupted in pathological states. In the healthy lung, oxygen in the alveoli diffuses across the thin cell membrane of a type I pneumocyte, through the interstitium, then through the endothelium of the capillaries into bloodstream.[5] Any disease process that interferes with these surfaces increases the diffusion time into the bloodstream, which can lead to hypoxemia. Common etiologies of diffusion impairment include the acute respiratory distress syndrome (ARDS), pulmonary edema, and interstitial lung disease. In ARDS, the deposition of hyaline material in the alveolar space adds an additional layer through which oxygen must diffuse.[6] Similarly, pulmonary edema refers to deposition of fluid in the alveolar space. Pulmonary edema can be caused by increased hydrostatic pressure in the capillaries, decreased oncotic pressure in the capillary, or breakdown in the barrier between the capillary and the alveolar space.[7] Interstitial lung diseases, in a broad sense, damage the interstitium of the lung and decrease the ability of oxygen to diffuse across it. Common etiologies of interstitial lung disease include idiopathic pulmonary fibrosis and fibrosis associated with connective tissue disease.[8] Some interstitial lung diseases, such as pulmonary alveolar proteinosis, cause deposition of substances in the alveoli and cause hypoxemia by a similar mechanism as pulmonary edema and ARDS.[9] These processes can be overcome by increasing the fraction of oxygen in the alveoli, which will increase the diffusion gradient, and therefore increase the diffusion of oxygen into the bloodstream.

## *Ventilation/Perfusion Mismatch*

Ventilation/perfusion defects occur when there is inadequate interaction between the air in the alveoli and the blood that supplies them. This category has some overlap with the conditions discussed with those discussed above under alveolar hypoventilation. When blood passes through the pulmonary circulation without ever being exposed to oxygen, this is referred to as a "shunt", which will be discussed shortly. One of the most common causes of V/Q mismatch is COPD. COPD is a mix of two separate disease processes: (i) emphysema and (ii) chronic bronchitis.[10] In many patients, these two processes coexist. In the emphysematous portion of the lung, the alveolar architecture breaks down, and blood is unable to reach ventilated airspace. In areas effected by bronchitis, the alveoli are unable to ventilate despite often-adequate perfusion. Both of these processes contribute to hypoxemia.[11] V/Q mismatch can occur in pulmonary thromboembolism as well. Pulmonary thromboembolism occurs when a thrombus forms, usually in the deep veins of the lower extremities, and becomes lodged in the pulmonary vasculature.[12] Pulmonary embolism causes blood to redistribute from areas of high oxygen exposure to areas that are less well ventilated in a process that is incompletely understood.[13]

### *Right-to-left Shunt*

A right-to-left shunt is a more extreme version of a V/Q mismatch. In these conditions, blood passes through the lung without ever being exposed to oxygen, or it bypasses the pulmonary circulation completely. Blood that does not undergo gas exchange has the same gas content on systemic venous blood and will alter the gas properties of ventilated blood when they mix. A shunt fraction can be calculated by the following equation:

$$Qs/Qt = (CcO_2 - CaO_2)/(CcO_2 - CvO_2)$$

In the above equation, Qs is the blood flow through the shunt per minute, while Qt is total cardiac output per minute. Qs/Qt is the shunt fraction, which represents the portion of the total cardiac output that is composed of shunted blood. $CcO_2$ is the pulmonary end-capillary $O_2$ content, which is approximately equal to the $PAO_2$. $CaO_2$ is the arterial $O_2$ content, and $CvO_2$ is the mixed venous $O_2$ content.[14] The most well-known causes of a right-to-left shunt are the cyanotic congenital heart diseases. In these conditions, blood from the right side of the heart bypasses the pulmonary circulation entirely. Unlike most of the causes of chronic hypoxemic respiratory failure, these diseases cannot be overcome by supplemental oxygen because the blood never reaches the lung.[15] Other common causes of right-to-left shunts include hepatopulmonary syndrome, pulmonary embolism, and hyperdynamic causes of shock such as sepsis.

## CHRONIC HYPERCAPNIC RESPIRATORY FAILURE

### Physiology

Carbon dioxide is a waste product of aerobic metabolism. $CO_2$ is removed from the body by the lungs. $CO_2$ diffuses into the alveoli and is eliminated by respiration.

It reaches equilibrium across the alveoli almost instantly, so disease processes that effect alveolar gas exchange do not alter the removal of $CO_2$ by the body. As such, removal of $CO_2$ is more dependent on the mechanical process of ventilation and patency of the airway than on the process of gas exchange. Ventilation can be defined as follows:

$$\text{Minute ventilation} = \text{Respiratory rate} \times \text{Tidal volume}$$

Wherein respiratory rate is defined as the number of breaths per minute, and tidal volume is the volume of each exhaled breath. Decreasing the respiratory rate or the tidal volume will decrease the minute ventilation, which will lead to increased retention of $CO_2$. In a healthy state, the medullary respiratory center interacts with the chest wall muscles and diaphragm to alter the minute ventilation to maintain $CO_2$ homeostasis.

## Pathophysiology

Appropriate ventilation requires processes involving the CNS, peripheral nervous system, chest wall, chest wall muscles, diaphragm, and airway. As such, dysfunction of any of these systems can lead to inadequate ventilation, which leads to $CO_2$ retention. When this dysfunction leads to a $PaCO_2$ of greater than 50 mmHg, this state is considered hypercapnic respiratory failure. The disease processes that cause this can be divided by the portion of ventilation that they effect.[16]

### Central Nervous System

The CNS is intimately involved with the process of ventilation. It innervates the various muscles that keep the airway patent and provides the respiratory drive that stimulates the process. One common cause of CNS dysfunction leading to hypercapnic respiratory failure is head trauma. Head trauma can cause denervation of the muscles that are required to keep a patent airway.[17] When these muscles lose their integrity the airway closes. Without a patent airway, $CO_2$ cannot be ventilated and removed from the body. This situation is a common cause of patients requiring long-term intubation and mechanical ventilation.

### Chest Wall

The chest wall is composed of 12 sets of ribs and associated muscles, vascular structures, and integument.[18] The caudal portion of the diaphragm also contributes to the chest wall. During inspiration, the chest wall must expand to all the lungs to properly inflate. During expiration, the chest wall can provide additional force to propel air from the lung. Common diseases of the chest wall that can lead to chronic hypercapnic respiratory failure include spinal malformations, morbid obesity and trauma. Obesity is an increasingly recognized cause of chronic respiratory failure, and the cause of respiratory failure in patients is usually multifactorial. Obesity, can obstruct the upper airway and decrease respiratory drive, but it also decreases the ability of the muscles of the chest wall to properly function. Moreover, increased abdominal girth can reduce diaphragmatic excursion resulting in decreased tidal volumes.[19] If the body does not compensate with an increase in respiratory rate, minute ventilation will decrease and hypercapnia will ensue.

### *Neuromuscular*

Neuromuscular diseases that cause hypercapnic respiratory failure include diseases of the peripheral nervous system that decrease the ability for muscles to ventilate the lungs. These disorders have a wide range of pathological processes, and include conditions such as myasthenia gravis, critical illness polyneuropathy, and poliomyelitis, among many others. Myasthenia gravis is an autoimmune disorder characterized by autoantibodies to the nicotinic acetylcholine receptor.[20] These autoantibodies can interfere with innervation of diaphragm, causing decreased ventilation and concurrent increase in $CO_2$. Critical illness polyneuropathy and myopathy occur when critically ill patients undergo degeneration of nerve tissue and muscle tissue, respectively. It is theorized that the loss of a sodium channel underlies both of these processes.[21] All of these possible causes lead to decreased ability to ventilate the lung and remove $CO_2$.

### *Pulmonary*

Pulmonary causes of hypercapnic respiratory failure include common diseases such as COPD and asthma. These diseases cause hypercapnia by obstructing the airway, which prolongs expiration and decreases the ability of the lungs to remove $CO_2$. COPD includes a range of pathology including chronic bronchitis and emphysema.[10] Chronic bronchitis leads to mucus production and hyperplasia of the respiratory bronchi, which obstruct the outflow of $CO_2$. Chronic fatigue of the muscles of respiration contributes to this process. Typically, the kidneys compensate for this chronic hypercapnia by retaining bicarbonate. Asthma, which causes obstruction acutely, is more associated with acute hypercapnic respiratory failure.

## MANAGEMENT OF CHRONIC RESPIRATORY FAILURE

As with acute respiratory failure, the mainstays of therapy for chronic respiratory failure include supplemental oxygenation and positive pressure ventilation. Positive pressure ventilation can be further subdivided into invasive and noninvasive modalities. While the management of acute respiratory failure may necessitate immediate life-saving interventions, improved outcomes in patients with chronic respiratory failure can be evident over the course of months to years of treatment.

## Long-term Oxygen Therapy

Long-term oxygen therapy (LTOT) is the standard of care for chronic hypoxemia and likely improves survival for most patients.[22,23] LTOT may also improve quality of life[24] and reduce hospital admissions.[25]

Prior research regarding LTOT has largely been focused on managing chronic hypoxemia in COPD patients. Its utility in chronic hypoxemic respiratory failure due to other etiologies has not been well elucidated. Current guidelines recommend LTOT for COPD patients with severe hypoxemia despite optimal medical management. Hypoxemia is best determined by ABG assessment, ideally with two separate determinations obtained while breathing room air for 20–30 minutes. Indications for LTOT include a $PaO_2$ per ABG of less than 7.3 kPa (55 mmHg) or arterial oxygen saturation ($SpO_2$) less than 88%.[26] Further qualified indications include $PaO_2$ of 7.3–7.8 kPa (55–59 mmHg) in the presence of cor pulmonale or polycythemia (hematocrit >55%), as these are end-organ sequelae of chronic hypoxia.[27]

The goal of chronic oxygen supplementation is to maintain $SpO_2$ greater than 90%, including periods of sleep and with exertion.[26] If oxygen demand is acutely or temporarily increased (i.e., during a COPD exacerbation), an ABG should be repeated in 30–90 days for reassessment.[27] Supplemental oxygen use for a minimum of 15 hours per day is considered necessary to be effective.[28]

Home oxygen therapy delivery systems include metal cylinders with an attached regulator to modulate oxygen flow, as well as oxygen concentrators, which separate oxygen from room air and traditionally required continuous electrical power to run.[27] Mobile patients require portable oxygen devices, such as liquid oxygen containers, which are relatively lightweight and do not require electricity. More recent developments include home concentrators that fill reusable portable cylinders, as well as portable battery-powered concentrators. Efficiency is improved by utilization of oxygen-conserving devices which restrict oxygen flow to intermittent pulses, inspiratory demand with variable flow dependent on the duration of inspiration, or a hybrid of the two.[29]

Though oxygen is not flammable, it acts as an accelerant. Open flames, including matches, or lit cigarettes should be strictly avoided while using oxygen. Patients should be educated on the hazards of oxygen use and receive training on equipment.[30] Worsening hypercapnia due to excessive oxygen administration is another risk. This is primarily a concern during acute exacerbations of COPD, and the risk can be mitigated by titrating supplemental oxygen to a goal $SpO_2$ of 88–92%.[31]

## Noninvasive Ventilation

Noninvasive ventilation (NIV) provides respiratory support without the use of endotracheal intubation, usually by means of positive pressure (Table 4). NIV can be administered via several interfaces, including mouth or nasal pieces, nasal masks, or full face masks.[32] For chronic respiratory failure, it is utilized in patients with COPD, OSA or other sleep-disordered breathing, OHS and other chest wall disorders, or neuromuscular disease.[33] The two most commonly used modalities of NIV are continuous positive airway pressure (CPAP) and bilevel positive pressure ventilation (BPPV). A now uncommon modality of chronic NIV involves negative pressure ventilation.

### *Continuous Positive Airway Pressure*

Continuous positive airway pressure utilizes a constant level of positive pressure throughout the respiratory cycle. This pressure prevents the periodic collapse of airways in patients with sleep-disordered breathing such as OSA. In OSA, recurrent episodes of hypoxemia, hypercapnia, and sleep fragmentation are caused by nocturnal apneic or hypopneic events, which can be detected via polysomnography.[34] CPAP can be applied and titrated during polysomnography so that different interfaces (nasal vs. full face mask), air temperatures and humidification can be attempted to maximize efficacy and patient comfort. CPAP is first-line therapy in treating even mild symptomatic OSA. The benefits of CPAP in treating OSA are wide-ranging and include improvements in daytime somnolence, cognitive function, cardiovascular disease, and overall quality of life.[33]

Continuous positive airway pressure is also used in the management of OHS. Most patients with OHS have concomitant OSA, and CPAP similarly prevents nocturnal airway occlusions in OHS patients.[34] This leads to improved daytime hypercapnia, though CPAP may not be sufficient to resolve nocturnal hypoxia. Patients who continue to have episodes of hypoventilation/hypoxia per polysomnography while on CPAP are often placed on variable positive pressure ventilation, most commonly BPPV.

| Table 4: Noninvasive Ventilation Modalities | |
| --- | --- |
| Continuous positive airway pressure | Constant level of pressure is applied throughout the respiratory cycle |
| Bilevel positive pressure ventilation | Continuous positive pressure plus pulses of greater pressure during inspiration |
| Proportional assist ventilation | Automatically titrates pressure support with varying airways resistance to maintain a constant work of breathing |
| Negative pressure ventilation | Thoracic cavity is enclosed in a chamber into which air is pumped in and out, inducing respirations |

### *Bilevel Positive Pressure Ventilation*

Bilevel positive pressure ventilation devices like CPAP deliver continues positive pressure throughout the respiratory cycle and help to maintain airway patency. In addition, increased pressure is delivered during inspiration. The differential between inspiratory positive airway pressure and expiratory positive airway pressure provides a gradient that drives ventilation. BPPV is used primarily in managing patients with inadequate ventilation, including severe COPD, restrictive thoracic disorders, and neuromuscular disease.[33,35] It is also used in sleep-disordered breathing that is refractory to CPAP, including central sleep apnea that requires inspiratory support.

Though the delivery of inspiratory pressure is often triggered by the patient's inspiratory effort, some BPPV devices can be programmed with a "backup rate" to ensure that the patient receives a mandatory minimal respiratory rate or minute ventilation.[33] This may be required for instance in patients with central or complex sleep apnea. Chronic BPPV dependence may limit patient activity and mobility. However, highly portable BPPV machines are under development.[36]

### *Contraindications to Noninvasive Positive Pressure Ventilation*

Apnea and severe encephalopathy are widely considered to be contraindications to NIV, as ventilation remains largely dependent on the patient's respiratory drive. Placing a mask on patients with emesis or excessive secretions is ill-advised, as this may precipitate airway occlusion and aspiration. Positive pressure ventilation may increase intrathoracic pressure and affect hemodynamics, and it should be avoided in patients with hemodynamic instability, pneumothorax, or pneumomediastinum.[32,37] Similarly, NIV may be unsafe for patients with head injuries due to increases in intracranial pressure. Finally, an inability to properly fit the mask, i.e., due to oral-facial trauma would preclude NIV administration.

## Negative Pressure Ventilation

Negative pressure ventilation, once the mainstay of ventilator support, is now largely obsolete. As it requires that the thorax be confined to an enclosed chamber, it is cumbersome and debilitating. Patients with chronic respiratory failure who cannot tolerate other NIV may still benefit from negative pressure ventilation, although the number of patients using this modality are exceedingly rare.[37]

## Long-term Invasive Positive Pressure Ventilation

Invasive mechanical ventilation may be necessary for patients requiring prolonged respiratory support and for patients for whom NIV is either ineffective or

| Table 5: Common Features of Invasive Mechanical Ventilators | |
| --- | --- |
| Pressure control vs. volume control | Applies pulses of either a set volume of or a set pressure of air |
| Pressure support ventilation | Provides a set pressure with patient-triggered breaths |
| Assist control ventilation | Provides scheduled breaths at a set rate and supports additional breaths triggered by respiratory effort |
| Synchronized intermittent mandatory ventilation | Delivers a minimum rate of scheduled breaths synchronized with respiratory effort |
| Alarms and monitoring | Apnea/low minute ventilation, low/high pressure, low/empty battery, pulse oximetry, capnography, circuit disconnect |

contraindicated (Table 5).[38] Invasive ventilator modalities utilize endotracheal intubation, which generally necessitates tracheostomy when long-term ventilation is needed. The advantages of tracheostomy include fewer oral ulcerations, improved airway security, better patient comfort, facilitation of pulmonary toilet, and possibly less pneumonia.[39]

Indications for long-term invasive ventilation include neuromuscular disease, CNS disorders or damage, anatomical defects of the thoracic wall or airways, COPD, restrictive parenchymal lung disease, and sequelae of pneumonia.[38] Long-term ventilation is sometimes required after acute respiratory failure, following failure to wean from the ventilator and failed attempts at extubation. The modality and intensity of ventilator and other life support is generally determined by the severity of the patient's disease, regardless of the etiology of respiratory failure.

Ventilators can apply positive pressure in multiple ways. Ventilators augment the patient's intrinsic respiratory effort. This is usually achieved by providing a target volume or pressure of insufflated air in coordination with the patient's inspiration, or as a separate mandatory pulse. Positive end-expiratory pressure is often provided as well. A wide degree of variability is present in ventilator features, including ability to utilize pressure and/or volume modes, ramping up or down the rate of airflow, maximum oxygen delivery rate, and variable mechanical breath triggers.[40]

### *Home Invasive Ventilator Therapy*

Patients with sufficiently mild and stable disease may be candidates for home invasive ventilation. Though more cost-effective than prolonged inpatient care, home invasive ventilation requires an adequate home setting, effective caregiver support and training, and continued close healthcare support.[41]

All home ventilator devices should be equipped with back-up batteries, alarms, and safety systems, and they should maximize patient mobility. The degree of ventilator sophistication should be targeted to the patient's needs to maximize cost-effectiveness and ease of use.[40]

### Morbidity and Prognosis in Long-term Invasive Ventilation

Initiation and maintenance of long-term invasive ventilation portends a grim prognosis, particularly if undertaken after acute respiratory failure.[42-44] As there may be significant discordance between likely outcomes and patient/physician expectations, a realistic assessment of the risks and benefits should be undertaken prior to tracheostomy.[43] A model using age, presence of thrombocytopenia, and requirement of vasopressors or hemodialysis has been proposed to predict 1-year mortality in patients requiring prolonged invasive ventilation after acute illness.[45]

## CONCLUSION

Chronic respiratory failure, either hypoxemic or hypercapnic, can result from numerous common pulmonary diseases. It is important for physicians to recognize risk factors for the development of chronic respiratory failure in order to educate, diagnose, and manage patients appropriately. New technologies allow patients suffering from this condition to live longer, better lives. However, use of these technologies should be applied judiciously with patients' personal goals and preferences being paramount.

---

### Editor's Comment

*Chronic respiratory failure is respiratory failure that has occurred over a period of time and, therefore, it is compensated so that the pH is normal. Hypercapnic respiratory failure occurs when there is an alveolar hypoventilation. This may occur due to decrease in minute ventilation or an increase in dead space ventilation. Decrease in minute ventilation occurs due to a central cause or due to a disease outside the lung parenchyma (chest wall, neuromuscular, etc.). Here, there is hypercapnic respiratory failure but the alveolar arterial gradient is normal. In disease where hypercapnic respiratory failure occurs due to an increase in dead space, the alveolar arterial gradient will also be elevated. Because of the varying pathophysiology, there are a number of causes for chronic respiratory failure. The focus of treatment is to try and prevent the progression of the failure by treating the primary cause as much as possible. Also, supportive care in the form of oxygen supplementation and assisting ventilation by either noninvasive ventilation or invasive ventilation if needed is provided.*

***Randeep Guleria***

---

# REFERENCES


1.  British Thoracic Society Standards of Care Committee. Non-invasive ventilation in acute respiratory failure. *Thorax*. 2002;57(3):192-211.
2.  Roussos C, Koutsoukou A. Respiratory failure. *Eur Respir J Suppl*. 2003;47:3s-14s.
3.  Pellegrino R, Viegi G, Brusasco V, Crapo RO, Burgos F, Casaburi R, et al. Interpretative strategies for lung function tests. *Eur Respir J*. 2005;26(5):948-68.
4.  Coin JT, Olson JS. The rate of oxygen uptake by human red blood cells. *J Biol Chem*. 1979;254(4):1178-90.
5.  Borland CD, Cox Y. Effect of varying alveolar oxygen partial pressure on diffusing capacity for nitric oxide and carbon monoxide, membrane diffusing capacity and lung capillary blood volume. *Clin Sci (Lond)*. 1991;81(6):759-65.
6.  Ware LB, Matthay MA. The acute respiratory distress syndrome. *N Engl J Med*. 2000;342(18):1334-49.
7.  Gluecker T, Capasso P, Schnyder P, Gudinchet F, Schaller MD, Revelly JP, et al. Clinical and radiologic features of pulmonary edema. *Radiographics*. 1999;19(6):1507-31; discussion 1532-3.
8.  Gross TJ, Hunninghake GW. Idiopathic pulmonary fibrosis. *N Engl J Med*. 2001;345(7):517-25.
9.  Marshall BG, Wangoo A, Harrison LI, Young DB, Shaw RJ. Tumour necrosis factor-$\alpha$ production in human alveolar macrophages: modulation by inhaled corticosteroid. *Eur Respir J*. 2000;15(4):764-70.
10. Balkissoon R, Lommatzsch S, Carolan B, Make B. Chronic obstructive pulmonary disease: a concise review. *Med Clin North Am*. 2011;95(6):1125-41.
11. Rodriguez-Roisin R, Drakulovic M, Rodriguez DA, Roca J, Barbera JA, Wagner PD. Ventilation-perfusion imbalance and chronic obstructive pulmonary disease staging severity. *J Appl Physiol* (1985). 2009;106(6):1902-8.
12. Lapner ST, Kearon C. Diagnosis and management of pulmonary embolism. *BMJ*. 2013;346:f757.
13. Burrowes KS, Clark AR, Tawhai MH. Blood flow redistribution and ventilation-perfusion mismatch during embolic pulmonary arterial occlusion. *Pulm Circ*. 2011;1(3):365-76.
14. Cruz JC, Metting PJ. Understanding the meaning of the shunt fraction calculation. *J Clin Monit*. 1987;3(2):124-34.
15. Sommer RJ, Hijazi ZM, Rhodes JF. Pathophysiology of congenital heart disease in the adult: part III: Complex congenital heart disease. *Circulation*. 2008;117(10):1340-50.
16. Shneerson J. Hypercapnic respiratory failure: from the past to the future. *Thorax*. 2007;62(12):1024-6.
17. Haddad SH, Arabi YM. Critical care management of severe traumatic brain injury in adults. *Scand J Trauma Resusc Emerg Med*. 2012;20:12.
18. Evans KK, Mardini S, Arnold PG. Chest wall reconstruction. *Semin Plast Surg*. 2011;25(1):3-4.
19. Piper AJ, Grunstein RR. Obesity hypoventilation syndrome: mechanisms and management. *Am J Respir Crit Care Med*. 2011;183(3):292-8.
20. Drachman DB. Myasthenia gravis. *N Engl J Med*. 1994;330(25):1797-810.
21. Latronico N, Bolton CF. Critical illness polyneuropathy and myopathy: a major cause of muscle weakness and paralysis. *Lancet Neurol*. 2011;10(10):931-41.
22. Continuous or nocturnal oxygen therapy in hypoxemic chronic obstructive lung disease: a clinical trial. Nocturnal Oxygen Therapy Trial Group. *Ann Intern Med*. 1980;93(3):391-8.
23. Long-term domiciliary oxygen therapy in chronic hypoxic cor pulmonale complicating chronic bronchitis and emphysema. Report of the Medical Research Council Working Party. *Lancet*. 1981;1(8222):681-6.
24. Eaton T, Lewis C, Young P, Kennedy Y, Garrett JE, Kolbe J. Long-term oxygen therapy improves health-related quality of life. *Respir Med*. 2004;98(4):285-93.
25. Ringbaek TJ, Viskum K, Lange P. Does long-term oxygen therapy reduce hospitalisation in hypoxaemic chronic obstructive pulmonary disease? *Eur Respir J*. 2002;20(1):38-42.
26. Celli BR, MacNee W; ATS/ERS Task Force. Standards for the diagnosis and treatment of patients with COPD: a summary of the ATS/ERS position paper. *Eur Respir J*. 2004;23(6):932-46.
27. Petty TL. Long-term outpatient oxygen therapy in advanced chronic obstructive pulmonary disease. *Chest*. 1980;77(2 Suppl):304.

28. Katsenos S, Constantopoulos SH. Long-term oxygen therapy in COPD: factors affecting and ways of improving patient compliance. *Pulm Med.* 2011;2011:325362.
29. McCoy R. Oxygen-conserving techniques and devices. *Respir Care.* 2000;45(1):95-103; discussion 104.
30. COPD Working Group. Long-term oxygen therapy for patients with chronic obstructive pulmonary disease (COPD): an evidence-based analysis. *Ont Health Technol Assess Ser.* 2012;12(7):1-64.
31. Abdo WF, Heunks LM. Oxygen-induced hypercapnia in COPD: myths and facts. *Crit Care.* 2012;16(5):323.
32. Elliott MW, Steven MH, Phillips GD, Branthwaite MA. Non-invasive mechanical ventilation for acute respiratory failure. *BMJ.* 1990;300(6721):358-60.
33. Nicolini A, Banfi P, Grecchi B, Lax A, Walterspacher S, Barlascini C, et al. Non-invasive ventilation in the treatment of sleep-related breathing disorders: a review and update. *Rev Port Pneumol.* 2014;20(6):324-35.
34. Chanda A, Kwon JS, Wolff AJ, Manthous CA. Positive pressure for obesity hypoventilation syndrome. *Pulm Med.* 2012;2012:568690.
35. Müller-Pawlowski H, von Moers A, Raffenberg M, Petri M, Saalfeld S, Lode H. BiPAP therapy of respiratory disorders in patients with congenital neuromuscular diseases. *Med Klin (Munich).* 1995;90(1 Suppl 1):35-8.
36. Carlin BM, Wiles KS, McCoy RW, Brennan T, Easley D, Morishige RJ. Effects of a highly portable noninvasive open ventilation system on activities of daily living in patients with COPD. *J COPD F.* 2015;2(1):35-47.
37. Corrado A, Gorini M. Negative-pressure ventilation: is there still a role? *Eur Respir J.* 2002;20(1):187-97.
38. King AC. Long-term home mechanical ventilation in the United States. *Respir Care.* 2012;57(6):921-30; discussion 930-2.
39. Combes A, Luyt CE, Nieszkowska A, Trouillet JL, Gibert C, Chastre J. Is tracheostomy associated with better outcomes for patients requiring long-term mechanical ventilation? *Crit Care Med.* 2007;35(3):802-7.
40. Gregoretti C, Navalesi P, Ghannadian S, Carlucci A, Pelosi P. Choosing a ventilator for home mechanical ventilation. *Breath ERJ.* 2013;9(5):394-409.
41. McKim DA, Road J, Avendano M, Abdool S, Cote F, Duguid N, et al. Home mechanical ventilation: a Canadian Thoracic Society clinical practice guideline. *Can Respir J.* 2011;18(4):197-215.
42. Bigatello LM, Stelfox HT, Berra L, Schmidt U, Gettings EM. Outcome of patients undergoing prolonged mechanical ventilation after critical illness. *Crit Care Med.* 2007;35(11):2491-7.
43. Cox CE, Martinu T, Sathy SJ, Clay AS, Chia J, Gray AL, et al. Expectations and outcomes of prolonged mechanical ventilation. *Crit Care Med.* 2009;37(11):2888-94; quiz 2904.
44. Scheinhorn DJ, Hassenpflug MS, Votto JJ, Chao DC, Epstein SK, Doig GS, et al. Post-ICU mechanical ventilation at 23 long-term care hospitals: a multicenter outcomes study. *Chest.* 2007;131(1):85-93.
45. Carson SS, Kahn JM, Hough CL, Seeley EJ, White DB, Douglas IS, et al. A multicenter mortality prediction model for patients receiving prolonged mechanical ventilation. *Crit Care Med.* 2012;40(4):1171-6.

World Clin Pulm Crit Care Med. 2016;4(1):137-55.

# Nutritional Management in the Intensive Care Unit

Inderpaul S Sehgal MD DNB DM, *Navneet Singh MD DM FACP FCCP FICS

Department of Pulmonary Medicine, Postgraduate Institute of Medical Education and Research
Chandigarh, India

## *ABSTRACT*

The evidence available so far supports that the enteral route should be used for administration of nutritional supplementation. Conventional strategies for enteral feeding are preferred to parenteral nutrition or modified enteral feeding strategies since there is no clear-cut evidence that any of the latter two are associated with improvement in patient outcomes. Most patients in the intensive care unit can be and should be given enteral nutritional support though, even at its best, it cannot completely reverse or even prevent the adverse catabolic effects of critical illness.

## INTRODUCTION

Malnutrition arises from an imbalance between nutrient intake and nutrient requirements (Figure 1). Diseases especially critical illnesses are unique in that they can not only affect nutritional intake and requirements but also increase the nutrient losses (urinary, gastrointestinal, or from other sites). In fact, in majority of the malnourished critically ill patients, multiple mechanisms are believed to operate simultaneously (Figure 2). Further presence of malnutrition can hinder recovery and increase morbidity and mortality.[1,2]

## MALNUTRITION IN CRITICAL ILLNESS

### Prevalence and Epidemiology

The prevalence of malnutrition among hospitalized patients, including those in the intensive care units (ICUs), has increased steadily over the years because of

*Corresponding author
*Email:* navneetchd@hotmail.com

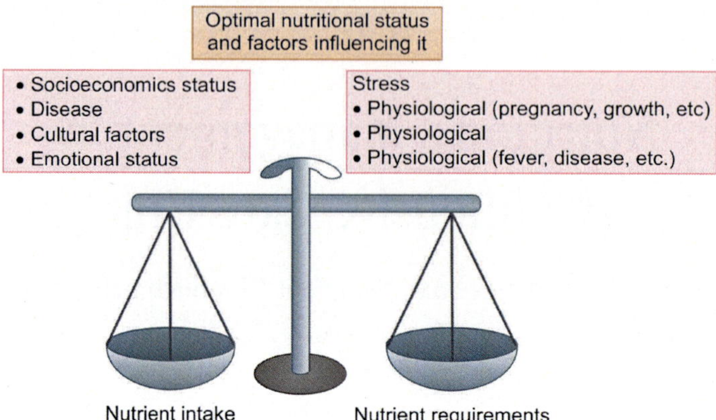



**Figure 1:** Factors influencing nutritional status and the balance between nutrient intake and nutrient requirements.

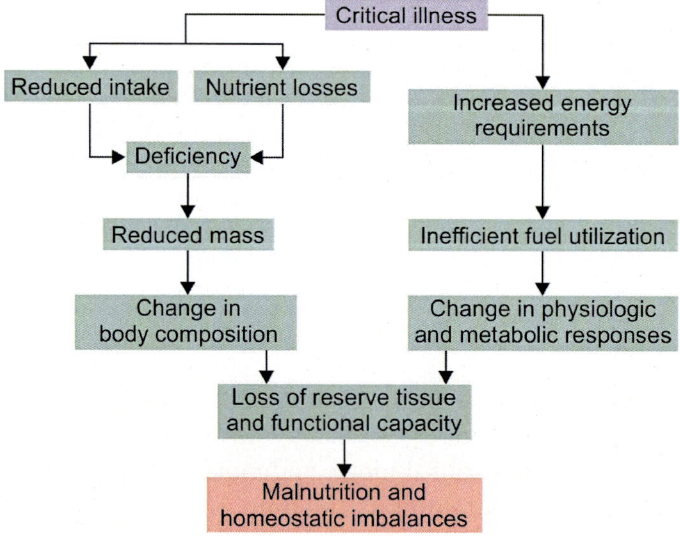



**Figure 2:** Mechanism of influence of critical illness on nutritional homeostasis.

several reasons including an increasing age of the general population, development of newer and often aggressive medical and surgical treatment modalities for different chronic debilitating diseases and finally progress achieved in intensive care management.[3,4] The prevalence of malnutrition among hospitalized patients is estimated to be as high as 30–50%.[5] Among patients admitted to the ICU, malnutrition is equally common, if not more.[6-8] Critical illness represents a continuum of four discrete phases: (i) acute critical illness (ACI), (ii) prolonged acute critical illness (PACI), (iii) chronic critical illness (CCI), and (iv) recovery from critical illness (RCI).[9]

Malnutrition can be either present on admission or develop subsequently as a result of metabolic response to injury. During ACI, myriad of endogenous substances comprising of hormones (adrenocorticotrophic hormone, catecholamines, glucagon, growth hormones, vasopressin, and others), cytokines, and chemokines that cause a shift from an anabolic state to catabolic state.[10] If not corrected it is succeeded by metabolic abnormalities, physiologic changes, reduced organ-cum-tissue function, and finally loss of body mass.[11] ACI is followed by a persistent proinflammatory state (PACI) representing contrasting physiology characterized by blunted hypothalamic-pituitary responses.[12] Some patients develop a chronic constant state of CCI, manifested by a paradigm of disease entities like kwashiorkor, marasmus, hypoproteinemia, hyperglycemia, immunosuppression, and neurocognitive dysfunction like delirium, depression, or psychosis.[13] RCI is marked by deliverance from mechanical ventilation and a return of anabolic physiology.[14]

Malnutrition can affect the pulmonary system directly by causing a reduction in diaphragmatic muscle mass, respiratory muscle strength, maximum voluntary ventilation, and functional residual capacity which make the process of weaning difficult. Optimal nutritional supplementation provides an opportunity to slow down or even halt the catabolic process and thus prevent malnutrition, which in turn can favorably alter the hospital course of such patients.

## Differentiation of Catabolism in Critical Illness from Starvation

It is important to differentiate catabolic state of critical illness from starvation. One of the fundamental differences between the two is that in the former the basal metabolic rate (BMR) is elevated while in contrast, it is depressed in the later.[15] Ketogenesis is a prominent feature of starvation but not critical illness.[11] Other characteristics of the catabolic process of critical illness in comparison to starvation are shown in table 1.

## Effect of Malnutrition on Clinical Outcomes in Critically Ill Patients

In some studies, the incidence of complications, hospital length of stay, and in-hospital mortality rates have been shown to be significantly higher in malnourished critically ill patients compared to those who are well-nourished.[6,8] Furthermore, presence of malnutrition has been shown to be associated with worse outcomes even with a lesser severity of critical illness.[6] In a prospective study conducted at

139

| Table 1: Differentiation of Catabolism in Critical Illness from Starvation | | |
| --- | --- | --- |
| **Feature** | **Catabolism in critical illness** | **Starvation** |
| BMR/REE | ↑ | ↓ |
| Respiratory quotient | 0.8–0.9 | 0.6–0.7 |
| Cytokine levels | ↑ | ↓ |
| Primary fuels | Mixed | Fat |
| Proteolysis | +++ | + |
| Ureagenesis | +++ | + |
| Urinary nitrogen losses | +++ | + |
| Gluconeogenesis | +++ | + |
| Ketone production | + | +++ |

↑, increase; ↓, decrease; BMR, basal metabolic rate; REE, resting energy expenditure.

the author's institute involving patients admitted to the respiratory ICU, mean daily calorie delivery of less than 50% of recommended values was shown to be independently associated with hospital mortality on multivariate analysis [odds ratio (OR) = 12.08; 95% confidence interval (CI) = 1.40–104.11].[16]

In several studies, no differences were seen between well-nourished and malnourished patients with regard to either length of stay or in-hospital mortality.[7] These discrepancies may be explained, in part, by the complexity of the relationship between the underlying conditions, which mandated ICU admission, and mortality.[17] Other reasons for such differences could be variations in the reported prevalence of malnutrition itself as a result of differences in type of screening tools used for its detection. Among the other clinically relevant outcomes, nosocomial infections have been shown to be more frequent in malnourished ICU patients.[18]

## REFEEDING SYNDROME

Refeeding syndrome represents maladaptive response to abrupt feeding after starvation and is characterized by dyselectrolytemia, respiratory failure, heart failure, and also lead to death.[19,20] Symptoms linked with increased risk for refeeding include one or more of unintentional weight loss of >15% within previous 3–6 months, body mass index of <16, inadequate nutrition intake of >10 days, low potassium, and phosphate magnesium before feeding, and two or more of body mass index <18.5, unintentional weight loss >10% in 3–6 months, little or no nutrient intake for >5 days, and history of chronic drug use like insulin, diuretics, antacids, and others.[19] It is important to recognize refeeding syndrome as it has been associated with higher risk of cardiac arrhythmias, heart failure, respiratory failure, and difficult weaning.[21]

## ASSESSMENT OF NUTRITIONAL STATUS IN CRITICALLY ILL PATIENTS

Assessment of nutritional status includes evaluation of clinical, anthropometric, chemical, and immunologic parameters. All the tests used for assessment of nutritional status have their own limitations and hence there is no single test that is sensitive and specific enough on its own to detect malnutrition in critically ill patients.[22]

### Body Weight

Alteration of nutritional status and protein calorie malnutrition is usually accompanied by weight loss. Unintentional loss of body weight (>10% in 6 months or >5% in 1 month) is clinically significant and suggestive of malnutrition.[23] Critically ill patients are often edematous due to progressive retention of salt and water, and in such cases, body weight may not reflect the actual body cell mass.

### Anthropometry

Anthropometric measurements provide an objective evaluation of fat and lean body mass. They are safe, simple, as well as inexpensive and can be readily performed at the bedside of patients including critically ill patients. Body fat reserve and skeletal muscle mass can be assessed by carrying out measurements of skinfold thickness (SFT) and midarm muscle circumference, respectively.[24] Measurement of SFT is based on the assumption that almost half of the total body fat is distributed in the subcutaneous region but this can vary from 20–70% in normal subjects.

Commonly, triceps SFT is measured but subscapular, iliac crest, and upper thigh are other areas that can be utilized. The normal values of these anthropometric measurements vary with age and gender.[25] There is also a tendency for over and underestimation of body fat in malnourished and obese patients, respectively. Fluid shifts that occur acutely in critically patients especially those who receive aggressive fluid resuscitation may alter the reliability of these measurements.[22,23]

### Hepatic Secretory Proteins

Albumin, prealbumin, transferrin, retinol-binding protein, and other proteins secreted by liver are used as indicators of nutritional status since they reflect visceral protein stores.[26] Since hepatic synthesis of these proteins is reduced in cases of acute infection/inflammation, they are referred to as negative acute phase reactant proteins. These proteins have different half-lives and their serum levels are influenced by factors other than nutritional status such as abnormal hepatic function, hydration status, protein-losing diseases, and acute infection/inflammation.[22,27,28] Despite the limitations, one or more of these proteins continue to be used for predicting patient outcomes.[29,30] In the author's experience, higher baseline serum albumin levels are observed among critically ill patients who survive as compared to nonsurvivors.[16]

## Other Parameters

The other parameters that have been used for nutritional assessment include total lymphocyte count and delayed cutaneous hypersensitivity.[31] Blood/serum levels of electrolytes like potassium, phosphorus, calcium, and magnesium are useful markers of adequate supplementation and these key electrolytes should be monitored with a frequency that depends upon the anticipated abnormalities, if any, in their levels.

## Multiparameter Nutritional Indices

These have been used to overcome the sensitivity and specificity problems associated with single nutritional assessment tests. Examples include Subjective Global Assessment, Prognostic Nutritional Index, and Prognostic Inflammatory and Nutritional Index.[7] However, even though these multiparameter indices are objectively designed, they again rely on the values of different clinical and laboratory parameters and hence are limited by the same concerns as the individual parameters themselves.

## GOALS AND PRINCIPLES OF NUTRITIONAL SUPPORT

General goals of providing nutritional support to critically ill patients include:

- Provision of nutritional support to the patient after taking into consideration his/her:
  - Medical condition
  - Nutritional status
  - Existing metabolic requirements
  - Route available for administration of nutrients
- Prevention (if possible) of nutrient deficiencies (both macro and micro) and treatment of existing ones
- Avoidance of complications associated with nutritional support (enteral and/or parenteral)
- Improvement in patient outcomes related to disease morbidity.

## TIMING OF INITIATION OF NUTRITIONAL SUPPORT

The timing of initiation of nutritional support has been an area of intense debate. Nutritional support is indicated in any critically ill patient who suffers from malnutrition (of any etiology) and is unable to eat. Many patients, especially those who are previously well-nourished, can tolerate short periods of starvation (usually <1 week) during a critical illness. However, even in well-nourished patients, nutritional supplementation is necessary if they are unable to resume oral nutrition or if their oral intake is insufficient for more than 3–4 days.[3]

Early institution (within 24 hours of admission) of enteric feed has been shown to have beneficial effects on the intestinal epithelium. Enteral nutrition increases the intestinal oxygen demand, hence causing concerns regarding its use in hemodynamically unstable patients. Current evidence suggests that early institution of enteral feed in unstable patients also increases intestinal blood flow and improves intestinal function, and may protect against bowel-related complications.[32,33] Though the evidence favoring use of target enteral nutrition in hemodynamically unstable patients is lacking, providing trophic feeds in this subset of patients may be beneficial and strike a balance between benefits of using the gut while reducing the risk of providing enteral nutrition.[34]

A delay in provision of nutrition in the presence of a hypercatabolic state, even for a short period of time, is likely to be associated with increased morbidity and mortality. Enteral nutritional support can thus be started as early as 12–48 hours of admission to the ICU. In most critically ill patients, oral feeding may not be feasible and hence enteral nutritional support should be attempted after placement of a nasogastric (or in some cases nasojejunal) tube.

In a retrospective analysis of a multi-institutional ICU database involving 4,049 mechanically ventilated medical patients, it was observed that 63% of the patients who had received early enteral nutritional support (within 48 hours of initiation of mechanical ventilation; early feeding group) had better outcomes compared to the remaining 37% patients (late-feeding group).[35] The early feeding group had lower ICU and hospital mortality rates (18.1 vs. 21.4%, p = 0.01 and 28.7 vs. 33.5%, p = 0.001, respectively). The lower mortality rates in the early feeding group were most evident in the sickest group as defined by quartiles of severity of illness scores. The early feeding group, however, had a higher incidence of ventilator-associated pneumonia (12.9 vs. 9.5%, p = 0.007). The authors had suggested that routine administration of early feeding might be warranted in medical patients receiving mechanical ventilation who are at high risk of death.

In a systematic review of 15 prospective randomized controlled trials (RCTs) involving a heterogeneous population of 753 adult ICU patients, effects of early enteral nutrition were compared to delayed enteral nutrition (initiation of nutritional support within and after 36 hours respectively).[36] Early enteral nutrition was associated with a significantly lower incidence of infections. Reduction in mortality in the early feeding group (8 vs. 11.3%) did not reach statistical significance. No difference was found between the two groups in terms of noninfectious complications.

A recent meta-analysis of 6 randomized trial initiations of enteral feed within 24 hours of hospitalization led to a significant reduction in mortality and a reduction in hospital acquired pneumonia.[34] Larger randomized trials are needed to demonstrate benefit of early nutrition as compared to delayed nutrition in critically sick patients.

## ROUTE OF ADMINISTRATION OF NUTRITIONAL SUPPORT

Nutritional support may be given by either the enteral or the parenteral route or both. There is increasing evidence to suggest that, in the presence of a functional gut, nutrition should be administered by the enteral route whenever possible. It is also becoming quite clear that the consequences of enteral nutrition go beyond the supply of nutrients to the body.[37] Modulation of the host's immune response and the provision of energy and protein to maintain gut integrity could be some of the possible reasons for the same. Enteral nutrition favors maintenance of structure and functioning of intestinal villi (both by reducing the incidence of mucosal atrophy as well decreasing the abnormal increase in intestinal permeability) and thus promotes gut motility that eventually helps in initiating oral feeding.[38]

The proposed mechanisms for the beneficial effects of enteral nutrition on the gut include stimulation of epithelial cell metabolism by direct contact with nutrients, increase in mucosal blood flow, and secretion of immunoglobulin A, and enterotrophic hormones like gastrin and enteroglucagon. Lack of enteral nutrition leads to atrophy of intestinal villi, bacterial overgrowth and increases permeability of the gut mucosa causing bacterial translocation. Provision of parenteral nutrition leads to a rapid atrophy of gut mucosa, it also impairs both humoral as well as cellular immunity.[39] Parenteral nutrition also leads to increased free radical formation, thus causing further damage. In addition to being more physiological, enteral nutrition is also less expensive. It leads to improved utilization of nutrients, and possibly helps to avoid some of the infectious complications associated with parenteral nutrition, one of the mechanisms being reduction in translocation of bacteria from the gut.[40]

## Comparison of Enteral Nutrition with Parenteral Nutrition—Evidence

In a recent EPaNIC trial, early (within 48 hours) initiation of parenteral nutrition (European guidelines, n = 2,312) was compared with late (later than 48 hours) initiation (American and Canadian guidelines, n = 2,328) in critically ill adult patients (n = 4,640) admitted in the ICU. Early initiation of parenteral nutrition was associated with worse clinical outcomes (hospital discharge, hospital-associated infection, days on mechanical ventilation, need for renal replacement therapy).[41] In the *post hoc* analysis of the EPaNIC trial, it was further demonstrated that the deleterious effects of parenteral nutrition were seen across all the groups irrespective of the severity of illness and the quantity of nutrition prescribed.[42] In a meta-analysis based on intention to treat principle of 11 trials that had compared enteral to parenteral nutrition in critically ill patients, a mortality benefit was seen in favor of use of parenteral nutrition.[43]

Another systematic review of 13 RCTs compared enteral and parenteral nutritional support in terms of outcome of critically ill adult patients. It included a heterogeneous population of 807 ICU patients.[44] Use of enteral nutrition in comparison to parenteral nutrition was associated with significant reduction in the incidence of infectious complications [risk ratio (RR) = 0.64, 95% confidence interval (CI) = 0.47–0.87, p = 0.004] as well as reduction in cost of nutritional support. There was no difference in mortality, duration of mechanical ventilation, or hospital length of stay. Moreover, use of parenteral nutrition was associated with increase in the incidence of hyperglycemia in addition to the total calories administered. This analysis again showed that enteral nutrition should remain the first choice for nutritional support in the critically ill.

The focus on another meta-analysis was on the comparison of early enteral nutrition with early parenteral nutrition among hospitalized patients. This involved 30 RCTs and included 2,430 critically ill medical, surgical, and trauma patients.[45] The definition of early enteral or parenteral nutrition used herein was the institution of supplemental nutrition within 96 hours of hospitalization, ICU admission, or surgery. No significant difference was found between the groups receiving early enteral and early parenteral nutrition in terms of hospital mortality. The results held true even when subgroup analysis was carried out separately for medical, surgical, and trauma patients. Use of parenteral nutrition was associated with an increased incidence of infective (including catheter-related bloodstream infections) and noninfective complications as well as prolongation of length of stay in the hospital. Importantly, among medical patients, in addition to the above, technical complications were also observed to be more frequent with use of parenteral nutrition. The only complication that was observed to be higher with use of enteral nutrition was incidence of diarrhea. Thus, even though no mortality benefit was shown in this analysis, enteral nutrition was shown to have significantly less complications as compared to parenteral nutrition in the setting of early initiation of nutritional support.

There is no denying the fact that parenteral nutrition remains a valuable yet challenging weapon in our therapeutic armory in the presence of gastrointestinal feed intolerance or failure. It should be used wisely and not indiscriminately because most intensive care patients with a fully functional gastrointestinal tract can be fed safely with enteral nutrition.[46]

## Addition of Parenteral Nutrition to Enteral Nutrition

There is a school of thought among intensivists that adding parenteral nutrition to enteral nutrition leads to improvement in calorie delivery and therefore may positively influence patient outcomes. Published literature seems to suggest otherwise.

A systematic review of five RCTs compared combined enteral and parenteral nutrition to enteral nutrition alone and included a heterogeneous population of 248 ICU patients.[47] In these studies, parenteral nutrition was initiated at the same time as enteral nutrition. There was no difference between the two groups in terms of mortality, rates of infection, hospital length of stay, and duration of mechanical ventilation. Combining parenteral nutrition to enteral nutrition leads to significant increase in the total amount of calories delivered as well as the total cost. This review again led to the conclusion that in critically ill patients who are not malnourished and have an intact gastrointestinal tract, starting parenteral nutrition at the same time as enteral nutrition provides no benefit in clinical outcomes over enteral nutrition alone.

## Contraindications to Enteral Nutrition

Enteral feeding remains the preferred route of administration of nutritional support in patients in whom there is no obvious contraindication. It is not uncommon to encounter absolute and relative contraindications for administration of enteral nutritional support. Enteral nutrition is absolutely contraindicated in patients with a nonfunctional gut due to intestinal obstruction, anatomic disruption, generalized peritonitis, or severe intestinal ischemia. Normally, splanchnic blood flow increases in response to nutrient load taken orally/administered enterally. This response is lacking in patients who have reduced gut perfusion due to severe or prolonged shock. Even if it occurs, it may not be sustained and this ultimately leads to hampered digestion and absorption. In fact, early feeding during hemodynamic compromise/shock can further contribute to mesenteric ischemia, infarction and even perforation.

It is prudent to withhold enteral nutritional support until hemodynamic stability has been achieved.[48] The fear of intestinal ischemia and necrosis during enteral feeding in hemodynamically unstable patients is refuted by studies demonstrating the rarity of such events.[49,50] Relative contraindications to enteral feeding include occurrence of abdominal distension while administration of enteral feeds, presence of localized peritonitis, intra-abdominal abscess or severe pancreatitis, patients with a terminal disease, comatose patients at high risk of aspiration, and patients with short bowel (<30 cm).[3,51]

## QUANTITY AND VOLUME OF NUTRITION SUPPORT

Recommendations and practice guidelines have been given and revised from time to time in relation to the quantity of nutritional support to be administered to critically ill patients.[3,48] These recommendations can be broadly discussed under the following subheadings.

### Energy (Calorie) Requirements

For most patients, provision of calories in the range of 20–30 kcal/kg/day is appropriate. Factors that should be taken into consideration while deciding the optimal amount for a given patient include gender, age, presence/absence of pre-existing malnutrition, type, and severity of critical illness as well as the phase of critical illness (acute vs. recovering). The target goals for energy (calorie) delivery should be determined at the time of initiation of nutritional support. It is desirable to achieve the goal of providing the entire energy requirements by the enteral route alone within the first 7–10 days of hospitalization.

### Protein Requirements

Protein delivery should be between 1.2–1.5 g/kg body weight/day (maximum 2.0 g/kg body weight/day). Patients with extreme protein losses (e.g., extensive burns, digestive or urinary losses) can be given higher intake.

### Volume Requirements

In general, approximately 1 mL of water is needed per kcal while administering enteral feeds. However, fluid requirements and restrictions vary from patient to patient and, therefore, the total volume to be administered may need to be individualized. The total amount of calories can be administered in a volume that is appropriate for the patient by changing the relative concentrations of the different constituents, namely, carbohydrates, proteins, and fats. It needs to be mentioned that the recommended proportion of carbohydrates, fats, and proteins is 30–70%, 15–30%, and 15–20%, respectively, of total calories.[3,22] For nonprotein calories, carbohydrates and fats should be in a ratio ranging from 1.5:1 to 2.5:1.

## Issues Related to Body Weight

Determination of body weight is an important issue for critically ill patients. It is neither easy to weigh patients in the ICU nor are such measurements free from errors since critically ill patients can have rapid and significant shifts in body water content. If direct weighing is not feasible, ideal body weight can be estimated from height and anthropometric tables. The body weight used for calculating energy and protein requirements often needs to be modified according to the baseline nutritional status. Malnourished and obese patients generally require calorie delivery based upon determination of an "optimal" body weight.

## Issues Related to Estimation of Energy Requirements

In addition to the simplified formulae given under the subheading Energy (Calorie) Requirements, more than 200 predictive equations (including the Harris-Benedict equation—the most well-known of all of these) have been published. By using the Harris-Benedict equation, the resting energy expenditure (REE)[52] can be calculated and subsequently the total energy expenditure (TEE) by multiplying REE with a stress/activity factor (normally 1.2–1.4 in critically ill patients). Indirect calorimetry is another method used for this purpose and is probably more accurate method than either the equations or simple formulae. Also, it is unclear whether patient outcomes will improve substantially if overworked staff and healthcare professionals in busy ICUs devote a significant percentage of their valuable time and effort in these calculations. Table 2 describes the important components of general care of the critically ill patient in an intensive care unit.

# DELIVERY OF ENTERAL NUTRITION AND ITS DETERMINANTS

The quantity of enteral feeds administered has been shown to be significantly lower than what is prescribed in as high as 40% of all hospitalized patients.[53] Other studies have shown that patients in ICUs also remain underfed.[54]

| Table 2: Key Components of General Care of the Critically Ill Patient |
| --- |
| • Hemodynamic and respiratory monitoring |
| • Judicious use of sedatives, analgesics and neuromuscular paralyzing agents |
| • Periodic assessments for weaning and tracheostomy |
| • Prophylaxis against stress-related mucosal disease |
| • Prophylaxis against deep venous thrombosis |
| • Glycemic control—avoid intensive insulin therapy |
| • Prevention of pressure ulcers |
| • Implementation of infection prevention strategies |
| • Avoid unnecessary transfusions |

In a prospective study involving more than 400 ICU patients, successful administration (defined as 90% or more of the prescribed value) was achieved in only 52% of the total (n = 3,526) feeding days.[55] Although the percentage of successful feeding days increased from 39% on day 1 to 51% on day 5, the overall average energy, protein, and volume intake remained 54%, 66%, and 75%, respectively, of the prescribed values. Feed intolerance was noted to be an important impediment to successful nutrition delivery. Use of formulations with a higher energy and protein density has been suggested to hence enhance the total nutritional intake.

## Prescription in Relation to Recommended Values

In a prospective study conducted at the author's institute, median calorie and protein delivery for patients admitted to the respiratory ICU were 55.1% [interquartile range (IQR) = 35.4–81.3%] and 46.7% (IQR = 31.6–72.1%) of the recommended values, respectively, on day one.[16] It is not just delivery that was suboptimal. Even the median prescription of calories and proteins was 88.9% (IQR = 80.4–99.0%) and 80.1% (IQR = 67.1–90.6%), respectively, of the recommended values on day one. The daily prescription and delivery of both calories and protein (as a percentage of recommended values) improved during the subsequent days of ICU stay (Figure 3). A similar trend has been documented in previously conducted studies as well.[56] It is important to note here that in our study, both prescription and delivery were lesser for protein in comparison to those for calories. Other studies that have compared actual prescription with recommended intake have also revealed protein delivery to be the area of largest overall deficit.

Feeding interruptions because of diagnostic or therapeutic procedures remain an important reason for this reduced intake. Other common reasons for decreasing or discontinuing feeds after initiation included high gastric residual volumes and mechanical feeding tube problems. Potential factors implicated for intolerance to feeds include the admission diagnosis, pre-existing illnesses, electrolyte and metabolic abnormalities, advanced age, and use of drugs (such as narcotics or catecholamines) and shock. Elevated plasma cholecystokinin concentrations have also been shown to correlate with feed intolerance.

## Position of Feeding

Adoption of a semirecumbent position while feeding patients is likely to have the best effect in terms of both tolerance to enteral feeds and patient outcomes. The frequency of clinically suspected and microbiologically confirmed pneumonia has been shown to be lower among patients fed in the semirecumbent position compared to those in the supine position.[57]

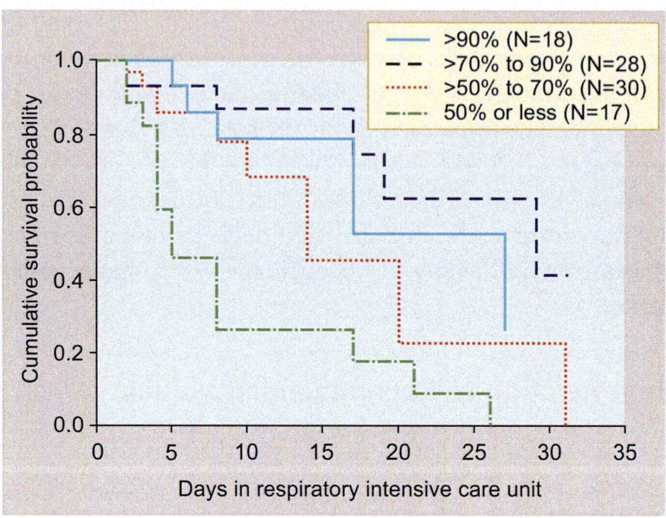


**Figure 3:** Kaplan-Meier analysis for probability of survival stratified according to mean calorie delivery (as percentage of recommended values). Mean calorie delivery of less than 50% of recommendations reduced the probability of survival significantly

## Nasogastric versus Nasojejunal Feeding

Nasogastric feeding is the most commonly employed method for administration of enteral nutrition in critically ill patients. Abdominal X-rays should be obtained, if possible, after placement of a nasogastric tube to detect any malpositioning (looping inside the oral cavity or in the lower esophagus, or introduction into the trachea). Nasojejunal feeding has been shown to be associated with improved tolerance of enteral nutrition, and, therefore, with a reduction in the requirement for parenteral nutrition.[58]

Although nasojejunal feeding leads to lesser gastrointestinal complications mainly because of a lesser incidence of high gastric residual volumes, it is also associated with increased frequency of tube-related complications (occlusion, accidental withdrawal, and dislodgment) and these can often negate its advantage(s) over nasogastric feeding. Moreover, in a prospective randomized trial, there were no differences between patients fed via the two routes in terms of feeding duration, length of ICU stay, and incidence of nosocomial pneumonia or mortality.[59]

Since nasojejunal tubes require endoscopic placement, use of this method, as is followed at the author's institute, should be reserved for patients who are intolerant to nasogastric feeding and in whom the intolerance is associated with inadequate nutrient delivery.[16]

## Residual Volumes

Gastric residual volumes should be measured ideally prior to administration of each feed or earlier, if indicated. It is advisable to have minimal residual volumes (ideally <150 mL) in order to reduce the risk of aspiration of feed contents into the tracheobronchial tree. However, there is no "minimum" level of residual volume that can identify patients at risk for aspiration as was shown by a prospective study.[60] In this study, yellow microscopic beads were added to enteral feeds. Diagnosis of aspiration/regurgitation was aided by the fluorometric detection of yellow color in tracheal/oropharyngeal samples. It was observed that the frequency of aspiration and regurgitation did not change appreciably even if the residual volume increased from 0 mL to greater than 400 mL. Even when the residual volume was less than 150 mL, the frequency of aspiration was 23.0%. There was also no correlation between the frequency of regurgitation/aspiration and the incidence of pneumonia.

In the presence of high gastric residues, a reduction in the frequency and volume of enteral feeds may be necessary along with more frequent monitoring of gastric residual volumes. Prokinetic agents (metoclopramide, cisapride, or erythromycin) can be used to improve gastric emptying although the relative efficacy of one drug over the other or use of a combination versus a single drug is debatable.[61,62] In most cases, it is gastric motility that is hampered (gastroparesis or gastric atony) and true ileus (dilated and nonfunctional small intestine) is rare.

## Role of Bowel Sounds

Bowel sounds should not be used as a criterion to determine initiation or interruption/discontinuation of enteral feeding.[48] The reasons proposed are:

- They do not correlate well with gut motility in critically ill patients
- Bowel sounds are produced due to movement of air through the small intestine and require the presence of both gastric air and gastric emptying. Critically ill patients who have nasogastric tubes *in situ* may not have either or both of these and hence there may be minimal or no movement of air from the stomach into the small intestine and hence decreased/absent bowel sounds even in the presence of a normally functioning small intestine
- Most clinicians do not listen for bowel sounds for more than few seconds while one needs to listen for them for 2–4 minutes in each of the abdominal quadrants.

Passage of flatus or stool is also not required for initiation of enteral feeding.[48,63]

## Diarrhea and Enteral Nutrition

Patients on enteral nutritional support who develop diarrhea that persists for more than 3 days may need evaluation for *Clostridium difficile* infection after other common causes have been excluded since these patients are usually receiving broad-spectrum antibiotics. A decrease in the frequency and volume of enteral feeds may be required and in certain cases, transient use of parenteral nutrition may be needed to ensure adequate nutritional support. Administration of antidiarrheal agents or probiotics like *Saccharomyces boulardii* can be considered but are of unproven benefit.

## CONCLUSION

Optimal nutrition is an important component of standard care in ICU. Malnutrition (deficiency or excess) is associated with poorer outcomes in terms of in-hospital morbidity and mortality. In general, enteral route is the preferred route for administrating nutrition. Parenteral form of therapy is resorted to in patients who do not tolerate enteral feeding and every effort should be made to switch to enteral route for nutrition. Provision of nutrition to critically sick patients should involve a multidisciplinary team comprising of physician, nutritionist, and the nursing staff. Nutrition should be tailored for each individual based on the formula that is used at a particular center. It is desirable to achieve the goal of providing the entire energy requirements by the enteral route alone within the first 7–10 days of hospitalization.

### Editor's Comment

*Presence of malnutrition among hospitalized patients in the intensive care units (ICUs) is an important factor for adverse outcomes. On the other hand, there is significantly a high prevalence of malnutrition among patients being admitted in the ICUs because of several reasons such as higher average age of these patients in the elderly range, aggressive medical and surgical treatment modalities being done for different chronic debilitating diseases, and multiple comorbidities. Moreover, the stay in the ICUs gets frequently prolonged, therefore, depriving the patients of normal nutritional intake. Supplemental nutrition is, therefore, essential for good treatment results. Conventional strategies for enteral feeding are preferred for administration of nutritional supplementation even though the enteral feeding cannot reverse or even prevent the adverse catabolic effects of critical illness. There is no clear evidence to suggest that parenteral nutrition or modified enteral feeding strategies have any advantage except if the enteral route is not medically indicated.*

**Surinder K Jindal**

## REFERENCES


1. Stapleton RD, Jones N, Heyland DK. Feeding critically ill patients: what is the optimal amount of energy? *Crit Care Med*. 2007;35:S535-40.
2. Cartin-Ceba R, Afessa B, Gajic O. Low baseline serum creatinine concentration predicts mortality in critically ill patients independent of body mass index. *Crit Care Med*. 2007;35:2420-3.
3. Jolliet P, Pichard C, Biolo G, Chioléro R, Grimble G, Leverve X, et al. Enteral nutrition in intensive care patients: a practical approach. Working Group on Nutrition and Metabolism, ESICM. European Society of Intensive Care Medicine. *Intensive Care Med*. 1998;24:848-59.
4. Lerolle N, Trinquart L, Bornstain C, Tadié JM, Imbert A, Diehl JL, et al. Increased intensity of treatment and decreased mortality in elderly patients in an intensive care unit over a decade. *Crit Care Med*. 2010;38:59-64.
5. Lafrance JP, Leblanc M. Metabolic, electrolytes, and nutritional concerns in critical illness. *Crit Care Clin*. 2005;21:305-27.
6. Giner M, Laviano A, Meguid MM, Gleason JR. In 1995 a correlation between malnutrition and poor outcome in critically ill patients still exists. *Nutrition*. 1996;12:23-9.
7. Atalay BG, Yagmur C, Nursal TZ, Atalay H, Noyan T. Use of subjective global assessment and clinical outcomes in critically ill geriatric patients receiving nutrition support. *JPEN J Parenter Enteral Nutr*. 2008;32:454-9.
8. Middleton MH, Nazarenko G, Nivison-Smith I, Smerdely P. Prevalence of malnutrition and 12-month incidence of mortality in two Sydney teaching hospitals. *Intern Med J*. 2001;31:455-61.
9. Hollander JM, Mechanick JI. Nutrition support and the chronic critical illness syndrome. *Nutr Clin Pract*. 2006;21:587-604.
10. Vanhorebeek I, Van den Berghe G. The neuroendocrine response to critical illness is a dynamic process. *Crit Care Clin*. 2006;22:1-15, v.
11. Chiolero R, Revelly JP, Tappy L. Energy metabolism in sepsis and injury. *Nutrition*. 1997;13:45S-51S.
12. Van den Berghe G, de Zegher F, Bouillon R. Clinical review 95: acute and prolonged critical illness as different neuroendocrine paradigms. *J Clin Endocrinol Metab*. 1998;83:1827-34.
13. Fletcher SN, Kennedy DD, Ghosh IR, Misra VP, Kiff K, Coakley JH, et al. Persistent neuromuscular and neurophysiologic abnormalities in long-term survivors of prolonged critical illness. *Crit Care Med*. 2003;31:1012-6.
14. Schulman RC, Mechanick JI. Metabolic and nutrition support in the chronic critical illness syndrome. *Respir Care*. 2012;57:958-77; discussion 977-8.
15. Pingleton SK. Nutrition in chronic critical illness. *Clin Chest Med*. 2001;22:149-63.
16. Singh N, Gupta D, Aggarwal AN, Agarwal R, Jindal SK. An assessment of nutritional support to critically ill patients and its correlation with outcomes in a respiratory intensive care unit. *Respir Care*. 2009;54:1688-96.
17. Bourdel-Marchasson I, Barateau M, Sourgen C, Pinganaud G, Salle-Montaudon N, Richard-Harston S, et al. Prospective audits of quality of PEM recognition and nutritional support in critically ill elderly patients. *Clin Nutr*. 1999;18:233-40.
18. Lee S, Choi M, Kim Y, Lee J, Shin C. Nosocomial infection of malnourished patients in an intensive care unit. *Yonsei Med J*. 2003;44:203-9.
19. Boateng AA, Sriram K, Meguid MM, Crook M. Refeeding syndrome: treatment considerations based on collective analysis of literature case reports. *Nutrition*. 2010;26:156-67.
20. Miller SJ. Death resulting from overzealous total parenteral nutrition: the refeeding syndrome revisited. *Nutr Clin Pract*. 2008;23:166-71.
21. Byrnes MC, Stangenes J. Refeeding in the ICU: an adult and pediatric problem. *Curr Opin Clin Nutr Metab Care*. 2011;14:186-92.
22. Cerra FB, Benitez MR, Blackburn GL, Irwin RS, Jeejeebhoy K, Katz DP, et al. Applied nutrition in ICU patients. A consensus statement of the American College of Chest Physicians. *Chest*. 1997;111:769-78.
23. Chan S, McCowen KC, Blackburn GL. Nutrition management in the ICU. *Chest*. 1999;115:145S-8S.
24. Ravasco P, Camilo ME, Gouveia-Oliveira A, Adam S, Brum G. A critical approach to nutritional assessment in critically ill patients. *Clin Nutr*. 2002;21:73-7.

25. Physical status: the use and interpretation of anthropometry: report of a WHO Expert Committee. WHO Technical Report Series No. 854. Geneva: World Health Organization; 1995.

26. Nataloni S, Gentili P, Marini B, Guidi A, Marconi P, Busco F, et al. Nutritional assessment in head injured patients through the study of rapid turnover visceral proteins. *Clin Nutr.* 1999;18:247-51.

27. Don BR, Kaysen G. Serum albumin: relationship to inflammation and nutrition. *Semin Dial.* 2004;17:432-7.

28. Lim SH, Lee JS, Chae SH, Ahn BS, Chang DJ, Shin CS. Prealbumin is not sensitive indicator of nutrition and prognosis in critical ill patients. *Yonsei Med J.* 2005;46:21-6.

29. Sung J, Bochicchio GV, Joshi M, Bochicchio K, Costas A, Tracy K. Admission serum albumin is predictive of outcome in critically ill trauma patients. *Am Surg.* 2004;70:1099-102.

30. Yap FH, Joynt GM, Buckley TA, Wong EL. Association of serum albumin concentration and mortality risk in critically ill patients. *Anaesth Intensive Care.* 2002;30:202-7.

31. Slone DS. Nutritional support of the critically ill and injured patient. *Crit Care Clin.* 2004;20:135-57.

32. Revelly JP, Tappy L, Berger MM, Gersbach P, Cayeux C, Chioléro R. Early metabolic and splanchnic responses to enteral nutrition in postoperative cardiac surgery patients with circulatory compromise. *Intensive Care Med.* 2001;27:540-7.

33. Kompan L, Kremzar B, Gadzijev E, Prosek M. Effects of early enteral nutrition on intestinal permeability and the development of multiple organ failure after multiple injury. *Intensive Care Med.* 1999;25:157-61.

34. Doig GS, Heighes PT, Simpson F, Sweetman EA, Davies AR. Early enteral nutrition, provided within 24 h of injury or intensive care unit admission, significantly reduces mortality in critically ill patients: a meta-analysis of randomised controlled trials. *Intensive Care Med.* 2009;35:2018-27.

35. Artinian V, Krayem H, DiGiovine B. Effects of early enteral feeding on the outcome of critically ill mechanically ventilated medical patients. *Chest.* 2006;129:960-7.

36. Marik PE, Zaloga GP. Early enteral nutrition in acutely ill patients: a systematic review. *Crit Care Med.* 2001;29:2264-70.

37. Dominioni L, Rovera F, Pericelli A, Imperatori A. The rationale of early enteral nutrition. *Acta Biomed.* 2003;74 Suppl 2:41-4.

38. Zaloga GP. Parenteral nutrition in adult inpatients with functioning gastrointestinal tracts: assessment of outcomes. *Lancet.* 2006;367:1101-11.

39. Alverdy JC, Burke D. Total parenteral nutrition: iatrogenic immunosuppression. *Nutrition.* 1992;8:359-65.

40. Jolliet P, Pichard C, Biolo G, Chioléro R, Grimble G, Leverve X, et al. Enteral nutrition in intensive care patients: a practical approach. *Clin Nutr.* 1999;18:47-56.

41. Casaer MP, Mesotten D, Hermans G, Wouters PJ, Schetz M, Meyfroidt G, et al. Early versus late parenteral nutrition in critically ill adults. *N Engl J Med.* 2011;365:506-17.

42. Casaer MP, Wilmer A, Hermans G, Wouters PJ, Mesotten D, Van den Berghe G. Role of disease and macronutrient dose in the randomized controlled EPaNIC trial: a post hoc analysis. *Am J Respir Crit Care Med.* 2013;187:247-55.

43. Simpson F, Doig GS. Parenteral vs. enteral nutrition in the critically ill patient: a meta-analysis of trials using the intention to treat principle. *Intensive Care Med.* 2005;31:12-23.

44. Gramlich L, Kichian K, Pinilla J, Rodych NJ, Dhaliwal R, Heyland DK. Does enteral nutrition compared to parenteral nutrition result in better outcomes in critically ill adult patients? A systematic review of the literature. *Nutrition.* 2004;20:843-8.

45. Peter JV, Moran JL, Phillips-Hughes J. A meta-analysis of treatment outcomes of early enteral versus early parenteral nutrition in hospitalized patients. *Crit Care Med.* 2005;33:213-20.

46. Griffiths RD. Is parenteral nutrition really that risky in the intensive care unit? *Curr Opin Clin Nutr Metab Care.* 2004;7:175-81.

47. Dhaliwal R, Jurewitsch B, Harrietha D, Heyland DK. Combination enteral and parenteral nutrition in critically ill patients: harmful or beneficial? A systematic review of the evidence. *Intensive Care Med.* 2004;30:1666-71.

48. Martindale RG, McClave SA, Vanek VW, McCarthy M, Roberts P, Taylor B, et al. Guidelines for the provision and assessment of nutrition support therapy in the adult critically ill patient: Society of Critical Care

Medicine and American Society for Parenteral and Enteral Nutrition: Executive Summary. *Crit Care Med.* 2009;37:1757-61.

49. Mancl EE, Muzevich KM. Tolerability and safety of enteral nutrition in critically ill patients receiving intravenous vasopressor therapy. *JPEN J Parenter Enteral Nutr.* 2013;37:641-51.

50. Khalid I, Doshi P, DiGiovine B. Early enteral nutrition and outcomes of critically ill patients treated with vasopressors and mechanical ventilation. *Am J Crit Care.* 2010;19:261-8.

51. National Heart, Lung, and Blood Institute Acute Respiratory Distress Syndrome (ARDS) Clinical Trials Network, Rice TW, Wheeler AP, Thompson BT, Steingrub J, et al. Initial trophic vs. full enteral feeding in patients with acute lung injury: the EDEN randomized trial. *JAMA.* 2012;307:795-803.

52. Boyle M, Green M. Pressure sores in intensive care: defining their incidence and associated factors and assessing the utility of two pressure sore risk assessment tools. *Aust Crit Care.* 2001;14:24-30.

53. van den Broek PW, Rasmussen-Conrad EL, Naber AH, Wanten GJ. What you think is not what they get: significant discrepancies between prescribed and administered doses of tube feeding. *Br J Nutr.* 2009;101:68-71.

54. De Beaux, Chapman M, Fraser R, Finnis M, De Keulenaer B, Liberalli D, et al. Enteral nutrition in the critically ill: a prospective survey in an Australian intensive care unit. *Anaesth Intensive Care.* 2001;29:619-22.

55. Binnekade JM, Tepaske R, Bruynzeel P, Mathus-Vliegen EM, de Hann RJ. Daily enteral feeding practice on the ICU: attainment of goals and interfering factors. *Crit Care.* 2005;9:R218-25.

56. Genton L, Dupertuis YM, Romand JA, Simonet ML, Jolliet P, Huber O, et al. Higher calorie prescription improves nutrient delivery during the first 5 days of enteral nutrition. *Clin Nutr.* 2004;23:307-15.

57. Drakulovic MB, Torres A, Bauer TT, Nicolas JM, Nogué S, Ferrer M. Supine body position as a risk factor for nosocomial pneumonia in mechanically ventilated patients: a randomised trial. *Lancet.* 1999;354:1851-8.

58. Davies AR, Froomes PR, French CJ, Bellomo R, Gutteridge GA, Nyulasi I, et al. Randomized comparison of nasojejunal and nasogastric feeding in critically ill patients. *Crit Care Med.* 2002;30:586-90.

59. Montejo JC, Grau T, Acosta J, Ruiz-Santana S, Planas M, García-De-Lorenzo A, et al. Multicenter, prospective, randomized, single-blind study comparing the efficacy and gastrointestinal complications of early jejunal feeding with early gastric feeding in critically ill patients. *Crit Care Med.* 2002;30:796-800.

60. McClave SA, Lukan JK, Stefater JA, Lowen CC, Looney SW, Matheson PJ, et al. Poor validity of residual volumes as a marker for risk of aspiration in critically ill patients. *Crit Care Med.* 2005;33:324-30.

61. Nguyen NQ, Chapman MJ, Fraser RJ, Bryant LK, Holloway RH. Erythromycin is more effective than metoclopramide in the treatment of feed intolerance in critical illness. *Crit Care Med.* 2007;35:483-9.

62. Nguyen NQ, Chapman M, Fraser RJ, Bryant LK, Burgstad C, Holloway RH. Prokinetic therapy for feed intolerance in critical illness: one drug or two? *Crit Care Med.* 2007;35:2561-7.

63. Baudouin SV, Evans TW. Nutritional support in critical care. *Clin Chest Med.* 2003;24:633-44.

World Clin Pulm Crit Care Med. 2016;4(1):156-68.

# Interpretation of Arterial Blood Gases and Acid-base Abnormalities

Aditya Jindal MBBS DNB DM FCCP

Jindal Clinics, Centre for Interventional Pulmonology and Sleep Medicine
Chandigarh, India

## *ABSTRACT*

Acid-base and oxygenation abnormalities are among the most common clinical problems faced, both in routine medical clinics and in the intensive care unit. Proper interpretation and analysis of the blood gas report can lead to major changes in the treatment protocols and be life-saving for the patient. Metabolic disorders are due to primary changes in bicarbonate while respiratory disorders are due to primary changes in carbon dioxide. The clinical features of acid-base disorders are more dependent on the underlying clinical conditions rather than due the presence of acidosis or alkalosis per se. Generally, respiratory and metabolic acidosis share common clinical features as do respiratory and metabolic alkalosis. There has been considerable interest in evaluating the use of venous blood for blood gas analysis. Further work is however required before the venous sampling can be routinely recommended.

## INTRODUCTION

Interpretation of blood gas and acid-base abnormalities is one area where most medical personnel face problems. This is primarily because of the excessive technical jargon involved in the area. However, one has to make a distinction between clinically relevant analyses and basic pathophysiological processes. The purpose of this article is to introduce the relevant pathophysiologic principles and develop a systematic and stepwise approach for the analysis of acid-base disorders.

---

*Email:* adijindal@gmail.com

The amount of carbon dioxide ($CO_2$) in the body is regulated within a normal range by the respiratory system, so as to maintain the pH within a normal range. Any disease process leading to an increase in $CO_2$ will lead to an increase in $H^+$ and therefore acidosis, while conversely any decrease in $CO_2$ will lead to alkalosis. Protein metabolism, in addition to the formation of calories, also leads to the formation of acids, which are not removable by the respiratory system. Examples of these acids include hydrochloric acid (HCl) and sulfuric acid ($H_2SO_4$), which are also known as "nonvolatile acids". These acids are buffered by the renal system, which uses $NH_4^+$ to excrete these acid loads and regenerates bicarbonate ($HCO_3^-$) while doing so.

In a typical diet, there is an addition of net acid to the body. This includes exogenous and endogenous acid as well as loss of $HCO_3^-$ in feces. This acid is referred to as net endogenous acid production (NEAP). The kidneys maintain the acid-base balance by excreting acid, known as renal net acid excretion (RNAE). This acid is excreted in the form of $NH_4^+$ or as titratable acid, with the simultaneous generation of $HCO_3^-$ and urinary buffers. The acid-base balance of the body is maintained when the NEAP is equaled by the RNAE.[1] Any disease may impose various acid or base loads; renal and respiratory regulations usually minimize these effects.

## TYPES OF ACID-BASE DISORDERS

We have seen that interpretation of the Henderson-Hasselbalch equation leads to categorization of acid-base disorders as either metabolic or respiratory. Metabolic disorders are due to primary changes in $HCO_3^-$ while respiratory disorders are due to primary changes in $CO_2$. These may be further categorized as metabolic acidosis and alkalosis and respiratory acidosis and alkalosis. The normal ranges of the pH, $pCO_2$, and $HCO_3^-$ are given in table 1.

The pH is normally tightly regulated within the mentioned range. According to the Henderson-Hasselbalch equation, this means that the $pCO_2/HCO_3^-$ ratio should not change significantly, i.e., for a primary change in the $CO_2$ the $HCO_3^-$ would change in the opposite direction and vice versa. This is also known as a secondary or compensatory response. For example, if the $HCO_3^-$ decreases and leads to a primary metabolic acidosis, the $CO_2$ will also decrease in order to maintain a relatively constant $pCO_2/HCO_3^-$ ratio and thus the pH (Table 2).

| Table 1: Normal Ranges of the pH, $pCO_2$, and $HCO_3^-$ | |
|---|---|
| • pH | • 7.36–7.44 |
| • $pCO_2$ | • 36–44 mmHg |
| • $HCO_3^-$ | • 22–26 mEq/L |

**Table 2: Acid-base Abnormalities and Compensatory Changes Based on the Henderson-Hasselbalch Equation**

| Disorder | Primary change | Compensatory response |
| --- | --- | --- |
| Metabolic acidosis | $\downarrow HCO_3^-$ | $\uparrow CO_2$ |
| Metabolic alkalosis | $\uparrow HCO_3^-$ | $\downarrow CO_2$ |
| Respiratory acidosis | $\uparrow CO_2$ | $\uparrow HCO_3^-$ |
| Respiratory alkalosis | $\downarrow CO_2$ | $\downarrow HCO_3^-$ |

$HCO_3^-$, bicarbonate; $CO_2$, carbon dioxide; $\downarrow$, decrease; $\uparrow$, increase.

However, it must be remembered that in disease conditions the compensatory responses are never strong enough to completely correct the acid-base abnormality, but serve only to limit the change in the pH. The amount of compensation expected in response to any pH change can be calculated and compared with the actual change to have occurred.[2] One must also remember that respiratory compensation for primary metabolic acid-base abnormalities occurs faster (minutes to hours) compared to metabolic compensation for primary respiratory disorders (hours to days).

It is pertinent to add here that it is entirely possible for two or more separate acid-base disorders to exist simultaneously. These can be detected based on calculation of the compensation. As an example, a patient of chronic obstructive pulmonary disease may have both metabolic acidosis due to sepsis and a respiratory acidosis due to the underlying disease.

## Respiratory Compensation

Compensation by the respiratory system for metabolic acid-base abnormalities, as mentioned before, is prompt.[2] It is mediated through the peripheral chemoreceptors which are present in the carotid bodies.

### *Primary Metabolic Acidosis*

A primary metabolic acidosis will lead to a fall in the $HCO_3^-$ levels and a fall in the pH. In compensation, the respiratory system will increase ventilation and blow off $CO_2$ so as to limit this fall, i.e., respiratory compensation. The expected $pCO_2$ can be calculated by the following equations:[3]

$$\text{Expected } pCO_2 = 1.5 \times (HCO_3^-) + 8 \pm 2 \text{ mmHg}$$

$$\text{Or}$$

$$\text{Expected } pCO_2 = (HCO_3^-) + 15 \text{ mmHg}$$

If the expected $pCO_2$ is equal to the measured $pCO_2$, it means that the respiratory compensation is adequate; this is called compensated metabolic acidosis. If the measured $CO_2$ is more than the expected, it means there is an additional respiratory acidosis; this is called primary metabolic acidosis with superadded respiratory acidosis. If the expected $pCO_2$ is less than the measured, it means there is an additional respiratory alkalosis, and it is known as primary metabolic acidosis with superadded respiratory alkalosis.

### Primary Metabolic Alkalosis

A primary metabolic alkalosis will be associated with elevated $HCO_3^-$ levels. In compensation, the $CO_2$ levels will increase. The compensation can calculated as below:[3]

$$\text{Expected } PCO_2 = 0.7 \times [(HCO_3^-) - 24] + 40 \pm 2 \text{ mmHg}$$

Or

$$\text{Expected } PCO_2 = (HCO_3^-) + 15 \text{ mmHg}$$

Or

$$\text{Expected } PCO_2 = 0.7 \times (HCO_3^-) + 20 \text{ mmHg}$$

The calculations for metabolic alkalosis are not as accurate as in metabolic acidosis; however, they do give a general idea of the expected responses. If the expected $pCO_2$ is equivalent to the measured $pCO_2$, the response is known as a compensated metabolic alkalosis.

## Metabolic Compensation

Metabolic compensation to primary respiratory abnormalities is mediated by the kidneys. As mentioned earlier, the time course is somewhat delayed. However, this is also dependent upon the chronicity of the disease. For acute conditions, renal buffering may be start as early as 5–10 minutes while in chronic conditions buffering may take from 2 to 3 days and indeed may be continuous as the primary disease continues to worsen.[2]

Clinically, metabolic responses may be divided into acute and chronic—acute before the onset of compensation and chronic after the compensatory response is well established. The kidney generates this compensatory response by varying the reabsorption of $HCO_3^-$. The kidney responds more effectively over a period of time; therefore, the magnitude of the chronic compensatory response is always greater than that of the acute response.

### Primary Respiratory Acidosis

The metabolic response to a primary respiratory acidosis will be an increase in the $HCO_3^-$ levels. As mentioned in the previous sections, the expected response can be calculated and compared with the expected to determine the adequacy of compensation and also the co-existence of secondary disorders. The formulae for compensation are as follows:[2,3]

For acute conditions:

$HCO_3^-$ is increased by 1 mmol/L for each $pCO_2$ increase of 10 mmHg above 40 mmHg

Or

Expected $HCO_3^- = 24 + [(Current\ pCO_2 - 40) \times 0.1]$

For chronic conditions:

$HCO_3^-$ is increased by 4–5 mmol/L for each $pCO_2$ increase of 10 mmHg above 40 mmHg

Or

Expected $HCO_3^- = 24 + [(Current\ pCO_2 - 40) \times 0.35]$

### *Primary Respiratory Alkalosis*

As expected, the metabolic response will be a decrease in the $HCO_3^-$ levels. Also, this can acute or chronic and can be interpreted as mentioned under the other acid-base disorders.

For acute conditions:

$HCO_3^-$ is decreased by 2 mmol/L for each $pCO_2$ decrease of 10 mmHg below 40 mmHg

Or

Expected $HCO_3^- = 24 - [(40 - Current\ pCO_2) \times 0.2]$

For chronic conditions:

$HCO_3^-$ is decreased by 4–5 mmol/L for each $pCO_2$ decrease of 10 mmHg below 40 mmHg

Or

Expected $HCO_3^- = 24 - [(40 - Current\ pCO_2) \times 0.4]$

The expected compensatory responses are summed up in table 3.

## ANION GAP

The anion gap is a theoretical concept; it is a value calculated from the concentration of electrolytes in serum. It has been used in the differential diagnosis of acid-base disorders, especially metabolic acidosis.[4] The anion gap reflects the value of the unmeasured anions in serum.

| Table 3: Expected Compensatory Response to Primary Acid-base Disorders[2,3] | |
|---|---|
| **Primary disorder** | **Compensatory response** |
| Primary metabolic acidosis | • Expected $pCO_2 = 1.5 \times (HCO_3^-) + 8 \pm 2$ mmHg<br>Or<br>• Expected $pCO_2 = (HCO_3^-) + 15$ mmHg |
| Primary metabolic alkalosis | • Expected $pCO_2 = 0.7 \times [(HCO_3^-) - 24] + 40 \pm 2$ mmHg<br>Or<br>• Expected $pCO_2 = (HCO_3^-) + 15$ mmHg<br>Or<br>• Expected $pCO_2 = 0.7 \times (HCO_3^-) + 20$ mmHg |
| Primary respiratory acidosis | • Acute:<br>  ○ $HCO_3^-$ is increased by 1 mmol/L for each $pCO_2$ increase of 10 mmHg above 40 mmHg<br>  Or<br>  ○ Expected $HCO_3^- = 24 + [(\text{Current } pCO_2 - 40) \times 0.1]$<br>• Chronic:<br>  ○ $HCO_3^-$ is increased by 4–5 mmol/L for each $pCO_2$ increase of 10 mmHg above 40 mmHg<br>  Or<br>  ○ Expected $HCO_3^- = 24 + [(\text{Current } pCO_2 - 40) \times 0.35]$ |
| Primary respiratory alkalosis | • Acute:<br>  ○ $HCO_3^-$ is decreased by 2 mmol/L for each $pCO_2$ decrease of 10 mmHg below 40 mmHg<br>  Or<br>  ○ Expected $HCO_3^- = 24 - [(40 - \text{Current } pCO_2) \times 0.2]$<br>• Chronic:<br>  ○ $HCO_3^-$ is decreased by 4–5 mmol/L for each $pCO_2$ decrease of 10 mmHg below 40 mmHg<br>  Or<br>  ○ Expected $HCO_3^- = 24 - [(40 - \text{Current } pCO_2) \times 0.4]$ |

The total negative charge in human plasma must be balanced by the total positive charge to maintain electroneutrality. The total positive charge in the serum is the sum total of the positively charged ions and other particles in the serum. These include cations such as sodium, potassium, calcium, and magnesium as well as cationic proteins. As the contribution of the sodium ion to the net positive charge is significantly out of proportion to the other cations, only sodium is considered in the calculation of the anion gap. Similarly, the negatively charged particles include chloride, $HCO_3^-$, anionic proteins, inorganic phosphate, sulfate and organic anions. Only the concentrations of chloride and $HCO_3^-$ are considered in the calculation of the net negative charge. Thus,

$$\text{Total positive charge} = \text{Total negative charge}$$
$$Na^+ + UC = Cl^- + HCO_3^- + UA$$

where, UC = unmeasured cations and UA = unmeasured anions. Rearranging the above equation, we get:

$$Na^+ - (Cl^- + HCO_3^-) = UA - UC = \text{Anion gap}$$

So, the anion gap, while calculated from the concentrations of sodium, chloride and $HCO_3^-$ ions, represents the difference between the unmeasured anions and cations in serum.[5] Traditionally, the normal anion gap value ranges from 8 to 16 mEq/L. However, use of ion-specific electrodes has led to a decrease in the normal anion gap; it is essential for clinicians to know the normal range from their respective clinical laboratory.[6]

It is obvious from the above equation that the anion gap will change with either decrease or increase in the levels of the unmeasured anions and/or cations. The causes of increased or decreased anion gap are mentioned in table 4.

The anion gap needs to be corrected for hypoalbuminemia before using it to interpret acid-base abnormalities. Albumin is the major unmeasured anion in serum and hypoalbuminemia will therefore lead to the determination of a falsely low anion gap. This is especially important in critically ill patients in the intensive care unit because of the high prevalence of hypoalbuminemia. The equation for the corrected anion gap (cAG) is as follows:[6]

cAG = Anion gap + 2.5 [Normal albumin (g/dL) – Measured albumin (g/dL)]

The most common cause of elevated anion gap is metabolic acidosis. The anion gap can be used for the classification of metabolic acidosis and can also help in the differential diagnosis. Metabolic acidosis involves an increase in the acid load in serum. Addition or underexcretion of organic anions to serum leads to an increase in the unmeasured anion fraction in serum and further on to an elevated anion gap. However, some causes of metabolic acidosis are also associated with a normal anion gap. The underlying mechanisms are not entirely clear; however, it is postulated that the retention of chloride by the kidneys to maintain electroneutrality may be responsible (Table 5).

| Table 4: Abnormalities of the Anion Gap[4,7] | | |
|---|---|---|
| **High anion gap** | **Low anion gap** | **Negative anion gap** |
| Laboratory error | Laboratory error | Laboratory error |
| Paraproteinemias (usually IgA) | Monoclonal (IgG) or polyclonal gammopathies | Bromide intoxication |
| Severe volume depletion leading to hyperalbuminemia | Lithium, bromide, iodide intoxication | Multiple myeloma |
| Metabolic acidosis | Hypoalbuminemia, calcium, magnesium intoxication | Iodide intoxication |

IgA, immunoglobulin A; IgG, immunoglobulin G.

| Table 5: Causes of and Anion Gap in Metabolic Acidosis[4–8] | |
| --- | --- |
| **High anion gap metabolic acidosis** | **Normal anion gap (hyperchloremic) metabolic acidosis** |
| • Ketoacidosis<br>  ○ Diabetic<br>  ○ Starvation<br>  ○ Alcoholic<br>• Lactic acidosis<br>• Addition of anions<br>  ○ Methyl alcohol<br>  ○ Ethyl alcohol<br>  ○ Propylene glycol<br>  ○ Salicylates<br>  ○ Pyroglutamic acid<br>• Renal failure (both acute and chronic) | • Gastrointestinal $HCO_3^-$ loss<br>  ○ Diarrhea<br>• Renal $HCO_3^-$ loss<br>  ○ Type 2 (proximal) renal tubular acidosis<br>  ○ Type 1 (distal) renal tubular acidosis<br>• Renal dysfunction<br>  ○ Some cases of renal failure<br>  ○ Hypoaldosteronism (type 4 RTA)<br>  ○ Type 1 (distal) renal tubular acidosis<br>• Ingestions<br>  ○ Ammonium chloride<br>  ○ Hyperalimentation fluids<br>  ○ Rapid saline administration |

## Gap-Gap Ratio or ΔAnion Gap

The anion gap can be used further to detect the presence of additional acid-base disorders or triple acid-base abnormalities.[5,6] Patients of high anion gap metabolic acidosis may have superimposed hyperchloremic metabolic acidosis or metabolic alkalosis which can be detected by this ratio. The gap-gap basically a comparison of the change in the anion gap to the change in the $HCO_3^-$ levels which should normally be 1.

The gap-gap ratio or Δanion gap (ΔAG) is calculated as follows:

$$\Delta AG = \text{Measured AG} - \text{Normal AG}/\text{Normal } HCO_3^- - \text{Measured } HCO_3^-$$

where normal AG = 12 mEq/L and normal $HCO_3^-$ = 24 mEq/L.

In case of a high gap metabolic acidosis, the ratio should be 1, as the amount of fixed acid added to serum should be titrated by $HCO_3^-$. Therefore, the increase in fixed anion should be equal to the decrease in $HCO_3^-$. If the ratio is less than 1, it means that the $HCO_3^-$ has decreased to a greater extent than the rise in the anion gap. This indicates a co-existing metabolic acidosis, which is usually a hyperchloremic metabolic acidosis. This condition often occurs in diabetic ketoacidosis or sepsis, where the existing high anion gap metabolic acidosis is often complicated by a hyperchloremic metabolic acidosis due to excessive normal saline (NaCl) administration.

## ACID-BASE DISORDERS

The clinical features of acid-base disorders are more dependent on the underlying clinical conditions rather than due the presence of acidosis or alkalosis per se. However, severe pH changes will lead to clinical features that are independent and superimposed over that of the underlying disease. Generally, respiratory and metabolic acidosis share common clinical features as do respiratory and metabolic alkalosis.[9,10]

## Acidosis

Severe acidosis is considered to exist when the pH falls below 7.20. This can affect multiple systems including the cardiovascular, respiratory and others. The cardiovascular complications include decrease in the blood pressure and cardiac output, reduction in the arrhythmia threshold, decrease in the renal and hepatic blood flow and shift of blood from the peripheral to the central circulation. These effects, compounded by a decrease in myocardial contractility, predispose to pulmonary edema with even minor fluid shifts. Acidosis also promotes hyperventilation and dyspnea (known as Kussmaul respiration) and also the weakening and early exhaustion of respiratory muscles. The metabolic effects of acidosis include development of insulin resistance, inhibition of anaerobic glycolysis, increase in metabolic demands, depletion of adenosine triphosphate, and protein denaturation. Ultimately, severe acidosis may lead to mental obtundation and coma.[9]

### *Metabolic Acidosis*

The causes of metabolic acidosis have been mentioned earlier (Table 5). Metabolic acidosis may be classified into high and normal anion gap metabolic acidosis for purposes of differential diagnosis. The treatment of metabolic acidosis is mainly dependent on the underlying cause. However, in severe acidosis, alkali therapy may be given in order to temporarily increase the pH and prevent the development of the adverse effects of acidosis.

Acidotic conditions where the acidosis is due to the accumulation of metabolizable anions (lactic acidosis and ketoacidosis) need not be given alkali therapy till the acidosis is severe (pH <7.2). This is because the accumulated anions will be converted to $HCO_3^-$ ions in a few hours if proper treatment is instituted and the kidneys are functioning normally. However, in conditions such as hyperchloremic acidosis, renal failure and acidosis due to accumulation of nonmetabolizable ions (renal failure and toxin ingestion), where the conversion to

$HCO_3^-$ is not possible and regeneration by the kidneys is either limited or slow in onset, alkali therapy is indicated earlier.[9]

The most common compound used is intravenous sodium bicarbonate. The amount to be given can be calculated by the following formula:

$$(\text{Target } HCO_3^- - \text{Current } HCO_3^-) \times \text{Body weight in kg} \times 0.5$$

The amount to be infused is dissolved in saline (because the $HCO_3^-$ solution is hypertonic) and infused slowly over a period of hours. The target in case of acidosis due to nonmetabolizable anions is to increase the $HCO_3^-$ slowly to the range of 22–24 mEq/L, while it is to increase the $HCO_3^-$ to more than 10 mEq/L and the pH to 7.15 in case of acidosis due to metabolizable anions. The use of $HCO_3^-$ therapy has been associated with several complications such as fluid overload and pulmonary edema and paradoxical worsening of the acidosis due to conversion of the $HCO_3^-$ ion to $CO_2$. Although $CO_2$ consuming compounds such as carbicarb and tris-hydroxymethyl-aminomethane have been used to prevent the latter complication, they have not shown significant benefit in clinical trials.[9]

## Table 6: Causes of Respiratory Acidosis

**Acute**

- Respiratory center depression
  - Infection
  - Trauma
  - Drugs—opioids, general anesthetics, benzodiazepines
  - Stroke
- Airway obstruction
  - Foreign body
  - Aspiration
  - Laryngospasm
- Parenchymal disease
  - Acute exacerbation of COPD
  - Acute severe asthma
  - Barotrauma
  - ARDS
  - Pneumonia
  - Pulmonary edema
- Miscellaneous causes
  - Electrolyte disturbances—hypokalemia, hypophosphatemia
- Acute worsening of chronic causes

**Chronic**

- Neurological/muscular disorders
  - Stroke
  - Guillain-Barré syndrome
  - Myasthenia gravis
  - Muscular dystrophy
  - Poliomyelitis
  - Hypoventilation syndromes
- Parenchymal/airway disorders
  - COPD
  - Pneumoconiosis
- Chest wall restriction
  - Kyphoscoliosis
  - Ankylosing spondylitis
  - Obesity

COPD, chronic obstructive pulmonary disease; ARDS, acute respiratory distress syndrome.

### *Respiratory Acidosis*

The causes of respiratory acidosis are given in table 6. The division into acute and chronic is purely for the purposes of diagnostic simplification—it should be remembered that any cause of chronic respiratory acidosis may present acutely due to worsening of the underlying disease and other precipitating factors like infections.

In addition to the general symptoms of acidosis mentioned earlier, respiratory acidosis may have additional symptoms due to the accumulation of $CO_2$. In the acute setting, these include dyspnea, anxiety, confusion, psychosis, and hallucinations with progression to coma and acute respiratory failure as the final event. In the chronic setting, symptoms include sleep disturbances with daytime sleepiness, memory loss, personality changes, impairment of coordination, tremors, myoclonic jerks, and asterixis (flaps).

*Treatment*: the treatment is mainly dependent upon the acuteness of presentation and the underlying disease. Patients with rapid onset of respiratory acidosis may require admission in an intensive care unit with intubation and mechanical ventilation. Chronically acidotic patients need to be treated holistically, with realistic treatment end-goals and priority given to relief of symptoms. These patients may require long-term noninvasive ventilation, which dramatically increases the quality of life in some cases.

## Alkalosis

Both respiratory and metabolic alkalosis may present with similar clinical features. Mild alkalosis is usually asymptomatic; symptoms start to appear as the severity increases (severe alkalosis is defined as a pH >7.6). At this pH, arteriolar constriction occurs, which leads to restriction of cerebral and cardiac circulation. Cardiac effects include reduction in the anginal threshold and predisposition to refractory supraventricular and ventricular arrhythmias. These are more prominent in patients with underlying heart disease. Alkalosis is associated with electrolyte abnormalities like hypocalcemia, hypomagnesemia, hypophosphatemia, and hypokalemia. Additionally, there may be stimulation of anaerobic glycolysis with anion production, leading to an increase in the anion gap. Alkalosis also leads to hypoventilation, which though a compensatory response, may be life threatening in patients with inadequate respiratory reserve. Finally, the neurological compilations include tingling, numbness, paresthesias, tetany, lethargy, seizures, and mental obtundation progressing on to coma. These may be worsened by the associated electrolyte abnormalities.[10,11]

### Metabolic Alkalosis

The most common causes include vomiting and nasogastric aspiration. The treatment is directed to the underlying cause. Use of antiemetics in vomiting and proton pump inhibitors in cases of pronged gastric aspiration may be sufficient. Likewise, reduction in diuretic dose or addition of potassium-sparing diuretics may ameliorate the clinical condition. In severe cases, exogenous acid administration in the form of 0.1 N HCl may be required.

### Respiratory Alkalosis

Respiratory alkalosis is the most commonly encountered acid-base abnormality in humans, primary because of its presence in normal pregnancy and at high altitudes, situations in which it is physiological rather than pathological.

The treatment of respiratory alkalosis is primarily directed toward the cause. However, in cases of anxiety hyperventilation, distressing symptoms can be temporarily ameliorated by rebreathing into a closed bag in order to increase the $CO_2$ levels.

## ARTERIAL VERSUS VENOUS BLOOD FOR BLOOD GAS ANALYSIS

There has been considerable interest in evaluating the use of venous blood for blood gas analysis. The advantages include ease of sampling and less discomfort to the patient. Studies on this subject have shown a good concordance between arterial and venous pH and $HCO_3^-$ levels. However, the $CO_2$ levels were highly variable. Moreover, these observations are limited to normal individuals and not in disease states. Further research is needed before venous sampling can be recommended as an alternative to arterial sampling for blood gas analysis.[11,12]

## CONCLUSION

Acid base disorders are among the most common problems faced by medical personnel during the course of patient management. These conditions have a major impact on outcome over and above that of the underlying disease. Familiarity with basic principles and a stepwise and systematic approach are required for the proper management of these conditions. Any of the available methods of interpretation may be used, as none have demonstrated superiority over the others in respect to clinical management. With the advancement of medical science and continuing medical research, one can hope that further diagnostic and treatment modalities will become available for better medical care.

> ### Editor's Comment
>
> *Arterial blood gases (ABGs) and their interpretation have now become an integral part of all intensive care units (ICUs). ABGs are now almost essential for assessing severity of respiratory or metabolic disease. Whether it is to decide on noninvasive ventilation in chronic obstructive pulmonary disease or the $FiO_2$ need in severe hypoxic respiratory failure, an ABG is always needed. Also to assess response to therapy, an ABG is frequently repeated to look at $PaO_2$, $PaCO_2$, pH, or bicarbonate. Most patients in the ICU have at least one ABG every day. Proper sample collection is important as more heparin or an air bubble in the syringe may give a false value. In any ABG, the pH, $PaCO_2$, and bicarbonate are the most important values to be looked at. This helps in deciding the basic metabolic or respiratory abnormality and also whether it is compensated or uncompensated. One also needs to calculate the alveolar arterial oxygen gradient and the anion gap for a comprehensive interpretation and to pick up any hidden abnormality in the report. Although ABG interpretation looks difficult, once the basic physiology is understood, most reports are simple to analyze. An ABG should always be interpreted keeping in mind the patient's condition and previous reports if available. For internists, pulmonologists, and intensivists, it is important to be comfortable interpreting ABGs.*
>
> **Randeep Guleria**

## REFERENCES


1. Koeppen BM. The kidney and acid-base regulation. *Adv Physiol Educ.* 2009;33(4):275-81.
2. Adrogué HJ, Madias NE. Secondary responses to altered acid-base status: the rules of engagement. *J Am Soc Nephrol.* 2010;21(6):920-3.
3. Berend K, de Vries AP, Gans RO. Physiological approach to assessment of acid-base disturbances. *N Engl J Med.* 2014;371(15):1434-45.
4. Forni LG, McKinnon W, Hilton PJ. Unmeasured anions in metabolic acidosis: unravelling the mystery. *Crit Care.* 2006;10(4):220.
5. Kraut JA, Madias NE. Serum anion gap: its uses and limitations in clinical medicine. *Clin J Am Soc Nephrol.* 2007;2(1):162-74.
6. Kraut JA, Nagami GT. The serum anion gap in the evaluation of acid-base disorders: what are its limitations and can its effectiveness be improved? *Clin J Am Soc Nephrol.* 2013;8(11):2018-24.
7. Lee S, Kang KP, Kang SK. Clinical usefulness of the serum anion gap. *Electrolyte Blood Press.* 2006;4(1):44-6.
8. Rastegar A. Use of the DeltaAG/DeltaHCO$_3^-$ ratio in the diagnosis of mixed acid-base disorders. *J Am Soc Nephrol.* 2007;18(9):2429-31.
9. Adrogué HJ, Madias NE. Management of life-threatening acid-base disorders. First of two parts. *N Engl J Med.* 1998;338(1):26-34.
10. Adrogué HJ, Madias NE. Management of life-threatening acid-base disorders. Second of two parts. *N Engl J Med.* 1998;338(2):107-11.
11. Soifer JT, Kim HT. Approach to metabolic alkalosis. *Emerg Med Clin North Am.* 2014;32(2):453-63.
12. Kelly AM. Review article: Can venous blood gas analysis replace arterial in emergency medical care. *Emerg Med Australas.* 2010;22(6):493-8.

World Clin Pulm Crit Care Med. 2016;4(1):169-82.

# Intensive Care Unit Infections and Antibiotics

**Raja Dhar** MD MRCP MSc CCT FCCP

Department of Respiratory Medicine, Fortis Hospital, Kolkata, West Bengal, India

## *ABSTRACT*

Severe infections in intensive care unit needs emergent coverage with empiric broad spectrum antibiotics with a commitment to de-escalation once the offending organism is identified and the sensitivity profile known. The emergence of antibiotic resistance is highly correlated with selective pressure resulting from inappropriate use of these drugs. All efforts should be directed to the prevention of antibiotic resistance by pathogens because the antibiotic pipeline is dwindling and the number of multidrug drug resistant pathogens is increasing. The way forward would be when medical professionals join hands with policy makers, hospital administrators and patients to minimize antibiotic usage. A team approach which includes the physician, an intensivist, nurse, infectious disease specialist, and a microbiologist should join hands in implementing "packages of interventions or care bundles" rather than "single strategies" in preventing infections. The topmost priority should be given to the prevention of infections by adherence to strict measures of asepsis and hygiene.

## INTRODUCTION

Antibiotics are the most frequently prescribed drugs among hospitalized patients admitted to any intensive care unit (ICU). Programs designed to encourage appropriate prescriptions in healthcare institutions are an important element in quality of care, infection control, and cost containment. Recent literature is replete with examples of authors expressing their concerned about indiscriminate and excessive use of antimicrobial agents that promote the emergence of antibiotic resistant organisms.

---

*Email:* docaardee@yahoo.com

We are at the crossroads with antimicrobial resistance today. About two-thirds of cases of ICU associated bacteremia are caused by multidrug-resistant (MDR) or extensively drug-resistant bacteria.[1] The effectiveness of universal strategies based on hand hygiene and decolonization or active surveillance culture and contact precautions for control of MDR bacteria in ICU is unclear. India has emerged as a "world leader" as far as bacterial disease burdened is concerned. Hence it is implied that antibiotics will play a critical role in limiting morbidity and mortality in our country.[2] As a mark of disease burden, pneumonia causes an estimated 410,000 deaths in India each year[3] and it is the number one killer in children.[4] A significant percentage of these deaths could be avoidable if patients had access to life-saving antibiotics when needed. At the other extreme, antibiotics are often prescribed for conditions like common cold and diarrhea where other appropriate treatment (oral dehydration for therapy for diarrhea) could effectively manage the situation.

"Drug selection pressure" is the single most important factor in the evaluation of drug resistance in intensive care. The reason for this selection pressure is multifactorial. Even though the actual resistance is a medical problem, the factors that influence the spread of resistance are ecological, epidemiological, cultural, social, and economic. Every times we use an antibiotic, for whatever reason, the probability for spread of antibiotic resistance is increased.[5,6] Antibiotics are a limited global resource and the responsibility for maintaining its effectiveness for as long as possible, while endowing maximal health benefit is a shared responsibility for every nation in our world. Each nation has to adopt strategies and policies tailored to its own conditions.

## CARDINAL SYMPTOM OF INFECTION

### Fever

Fever should be considered to be significant in intensive care when body temperature is greater than 101°F (38.3°C) and a proper assessment should be carried out to make sure whether infection is present or not.

It is worth remembering that more than 50% of intensive care fever has no associated infection. Fever could be a sign of inflammation with no apparent infection hence noninfectious causes of fever must be ruled out before subjecting patients to costly antibiotics which could potentially worsen the resistance profile in a critical care unit.

Infectious causes of fever in ICU:

- Sinusitis
- Catheter-related bloodstream infection
- Ventilator-associated pneumonia (VAP)

- Catheter-associated urinary tract infection (UTI)
- Wound infection.

Noninfectious causes of fever in ICU:

- Postoperative fever: fever on the first operative day following surgery is reported in 15–40% of cases[7]
- Procedures: hemodialysis, bronchoscopy, blood transfusion
- Endocrine causes: thyrotoxicosis, adrenal crisis
- Myocardial infarction, stroke, and venous thromboembolism
- Drug fever, common offending drugs are cephalosporins, penicillin and amphotericin B and phenytoin.

## CURRENT SITUATION IN INDIA

### Rising Antibiotic Use

The overall sale of antibiotics has increased by 40% between 2005 and 2009. The most striking rise was in the use of cephalosporins in a 5-year period but some increase was seen in most antibiotic classes except with the use of macrolides[8] (Figure 1). Smaller retrospective studies done in tertiary care centers between

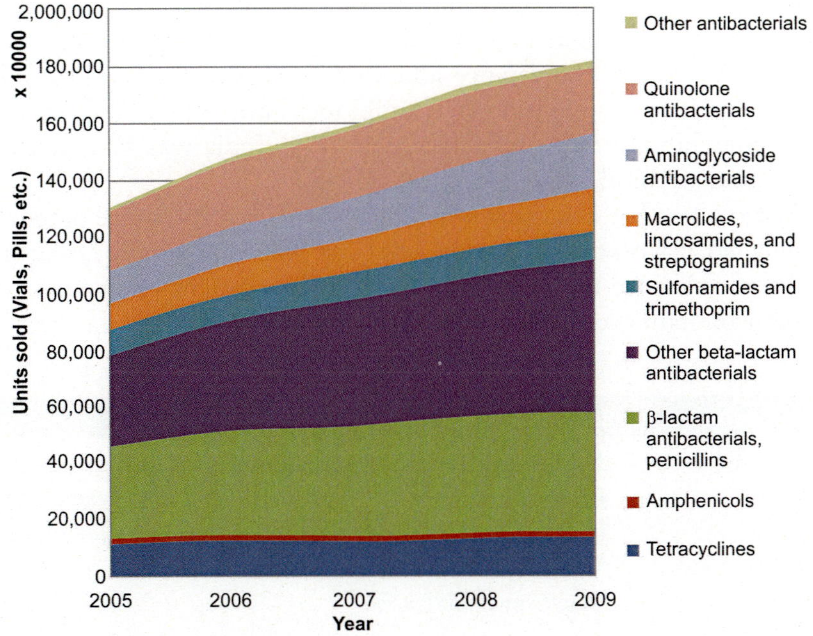


**Figure 1:** Units of antibiotics sold in India, by type.

2010 and 2013 show a fivefold rise in the use of carbapenems and in the last 2 years there has been a remarkable rise in the use of colistin in ICUs.

## Resistance to Antibiotics

In developing countries, the immediate challenges in healthcare would be areas like acquired immunodeficiency syndrome (AIDS), tuberculosis, malaria, pneumonia, and other infectious diseases. Antibiotics resistance would remain a relatively low priority area in countries like ours. In India, the issue came to fore when New Delhi metallo-beta-lactamase-1 (NDM-1), first reported in 2009, made front page news in 2010. The wide publicity about NDM-1 was due to a Swedish patient in whom it was first identified after he had undergone surgery in a New Delhi Hospital.[9] NDM-1 is an enzyme produced by the gene $bla_{NDM-1}$.[9] This gene was carried and classified and could be transferred between different bacterial species, in this case between *Klebsiella pneumoniae* and *Escherichia coli*, and most importantly, conferred broad resistance to most antibiotics, including carbapenems. The same bug was later reported from a tertiary care center in Mumbai.[10] Even though NDM-1 has got the most publicity in India, recent studies have shown significant rates of resistance to a wide range of antibiotics. The most prominent among these are hospital-acquired Gram-negative infections with *Acinetobacter*, *Pseudomonas*, *Klebsiella*, *E. coli*, *Salmonella*, etc. These are summarized in table 1.

A World Health Organization study in which *E. coli* was used as an indicator organism as four sites found high resistance rates in pathogenic isolates.[11] This study looked at antibiotic resistance and antibiotic use over 1 year at all these four sites. Resistance was highest when antibiotics have been used for the longest period of time. However, the resistance pattern in India was also adverse with relatively newer antibiotics like fluoroquinolones.

The bottom line has been that whenever studies and resistance patterns have been conducted, it has seemed that the levels are worryingly high. Unfortunately, these adverse resistance trends are affecting not just patient's outcomes but also result in concomitant economic adversity for the country.

| Table 1: Indications for Empirical Treatment | |
|---|---|
| **Clinical condition** | **Antimicrobial regimens (IV therapy)** |
| Immunocompetent adult | Piperacilin-tazobactam/meropenem/cefepime ± vancomycin |
| Neutropenia (<500 neutrophils/µL) | Piperacilin-tazobactam/meropenem/cefepime + aminoglycoside ± vancomycin |
| Splenectomy | Cefotaxime/ceftriaxone |
| IV drug user | Vancomycin |

IV, intravenous.

## Antibiotics Resistance Surveillance

There have been small scale efforts in India by the Indian Council of Medical Research and some pilot studies by private agencies. The Invasive Bacterial Infection Surveillance project produced valuable information on pneumonia in India even though it was a failure in establishing a permanent surveillance system for antibiotic resistance.[12]

### *Infections Acquired in Hospitals*

The greatest emphasis for infection control in the hospital is regarding hospital-acquired infections (HAIs). *Staphylococcus aureus* and *Pseudomonas aeruginosa* are the most common bugs for HAIs throughout the world. The studies conducted in India show a pattern which is generally similar even though the incidence of Gram-negative infection seems to be higher in our country and the incidence of methicillin-resistant *Staphylococcus aureus* (MRSA) is lower. A study by the International Nosocomial Infection Control Consortium (12 ICUs) in seven Indian cities followed 10,835 patients hospitalized for a total of 52,518 days. In this cohort, HAIs were 476 in number (4%). Of this, 46% were *Enterobacteriaceae*, 27% *Pseudomonas* species, 6% *Acinetobacter* species, 8% *Candida* species and 3% *S. aureus*.[13]

When we think about antibiotic resistance we can consider it in 2 different perspectives. We classify them as Gram-positive and Gram-negative bacteria and look at their resistance profile (Tables 2 and 3). We can also think about it in the context of site of infection in the body (Tables 4, 5, and 6). Aside from bacterial infection, the immunocompromised host can also suffer from hospital acquired fungal sepsis. The empirical treatment for this is outlined in table 7. The duration of antibiotic treatment is varies between 5 and 28 days and depends mainly on the severity and site of infections (Table 8).

## Patterns of Antibiotics Overuse

There have been a handful of hospitals and city based studies which have looked at irrational and inappropriate antibiotic usage in India. These medications are often prescribed at wrong dosage, frequency, and duration; hence patients suffer an increased number of side effects due to this irrational use. Over prescribing and overuse has been seen in all scenarios: public and private hospitals, clinics, and pharmacy. Approximately 45–80% of patients in India with an acute respiratory tract infection or diarrhea are likely to be prescribed an antibiotic even though it will not be effective in a viral illness.[14,15]

**Table 2: Treatment Options for Resistant Gram-positive Bacteria**

| Drug | Route of administration | Activity against MRSA | Activity against resistant *S. pneumoniae* | Activity against vancomycin-resistant Enterococci |
|---|---|---|---|---|
| Vancomycin | IV only | Yes | Yes | No |
| Daptomycin | IV only | Skin infection/ bloodstream infection | No | Yes |
| Linezolid | IV or oral | Pneumonia/skin infection | No | Yes |
| Quinupristin-dalfupristin | IV only | Yes | No | Yes, against *E. faecium* |
| Telavancin | IV only | Skin infection/ pneumonia | Yes | Yes |
| Tigecycline | IV only | Pneumonia/skin infection | Yes | Yes |
| Ceftaroline | IV only | Pneumonia/skin infection | Yes | No |

IV, intravenous.

**Table 3: Treatment Options for Resistant Gram-negative Bacteria**

| Organism | First-line therapy | Second-line therapy |
|---|---|---|
| • Empirical therapy | | |
| ○ Monomicrobial infection | ○ Carbapenem<br>○ Tigecycline (not in UTIs) ± antipseudomonal agent | ○ Piperacillin-tazobactam Colistin |
| ○ Polymicrobial infection | ○ Carbapenem + vancomycin<br>○ Tigecycline (not in UTIs) ± antipseudomonal agent | ○ Piperacillin-tazobactam + vancomycin<br>○ Colistin + vancomycin |
| • Directed therapy | | |
| ○ ESBL-producing Enterobacteriaceae | ○ Carbapenem Piperacillin-Tazobactam | ○ Tigecycline (not in UTIs)<br>○ Fluoroquinolone<br>○ Colistin |
| ○ Carbapenemase-producing ○ Enterobacteriaceae | ○ Tigecycline<br>○ Colistin | ○ Fosfomycin (parenteral formulation) |
| ○ MDR *P. aeruginosa* | ○ Meropenem | ○ Colistin |

UTI, urinary tract infection; ESBL, extended-spectrum beta-lactamases, MDR, multiple drug resistance.

**Table 4: Antibiotic Therapy Depending on the Site of Infection**

| Site of infection | Bacteria | Suggested treatment |
|---|---|---|
| UTI | *E. coli* | Ceftriaxone or ceftazidime ± aminoglycoside |
| Severe acute pyelonehritis | *P. aeruginosa*<br>*Enterococcus* species<br>*Staphylococcus* species | |
| Intra-abdominal sepsis | *E. coli*<br>*P. aeruginosa*<br>*Enterococcus* species<br>*Bacteroides* species | Ertapenem<br>Piperacillin-tazobactam<br>Third- or fourth-generation cephalosporin (active against *P. aeruginosa*) + metronidazole |
| Nosocomial pneumonia | *Enterobacteriaceae*<br>*P. aeruginosa*<br>*S. aureus*<br>*S. pneumoniae*<br>*H. influenzae* | β-lactam (active against *P. aeruginosa*) ± aminoglycoside ± glycopeptide (vancomycin) |
| Pneumonia without risk factors for MDR | *S. aureus* | Third-generation cephalosporin ± macrolide |
| *Pseudomonas* | *S. pneumoniae*<br>*H. influenzae*<br>*Other Gram-negative bacilli* | |
| Skin infections | *Streptococcus* species<br>*Staphylococcus* species<br>Gram-negative bacilli | β-lactam + β-lactamase inhibitor<br>Piperacillin-tazobactam<br>Carbapenem |
| CRBSI | *Staphylococcus* species<br>*Enterobacteriaceae*<br>*P. aeruginosa* | Vancomycin + β-lactam with activity against *P. aeruginosa* |

UTI, urinary tract infection; MDR, multiple drug resistance; CRBSI, catheter-related bloodstream infection.

The cause for this overuse is however more difficult to determine. The reasons might include a plethora of factors:

- Lack of microbiological facilities or unwillingness for the patients to undergo tests[16]
- A large number of doctors would take fever as being unequivocal evidence of bacterial infection and hence prescribe antibiotics
- Doctors often end up satisfying the patient's expectations of being prescribed antibiotic in an outpatient department[16,17]
- Patients replicating a previous doctor's prescription by buying the drug over the counter
- The pharmacist's incentive for selling antibiotics and other drugs over the counter[18,19]
- The public's lack of knowledge about appropriate use of antibiotics [Global Antibiotic Resistance Partnership-India].[16,20,21]

**Table 5: Management of Respiratory Tract: Aspiration Pneumonia (e.g., Post-cardiac Arrest)**

| Regimen | Drug | Dose |
|---|---|---|
| • In patients with immediate penicilline hypersensitivity as single agent use either | • Benzylpencillin<br>• Metronidazole<br><br>or<br><br>• Lincomycin or<br>• Clindamycin | • 1.2 g IV hourly<br>• 500 mg IV 12 hourly<br><br><br><br>• 600 mg IV 8 hourly<br>• 450 mg IV 8 hourly |
| **Special circumatances** | | |
| • In patients where aerobic Gram-negatives are suspicted (e.g., in alcoholic patient) add (recommendation by QUAIC Excpert Advisory Group not Antibiotic Guidelines 14) | • Gentamicin | • 4–6 mg/kg (severe sepsis: 7 mg/kg) for 1 dose, then determine dosing interval for a mazimum of either 1 or 2 further doses based on renal dunction (see Tables 1 and 2) |
| • In patients with known or suspected pseudomonal pneumonia (e.g., bronchiectasis with past pseudomonal colonisation) NB1 | • Piperacillin/ tazobactam<br><br>• Gentamicin | • 4 + 0.5 g IV 6 hourly<br><br><br>• 4–6 mg/kg (severe sepsis: 7 mg/kg) for 1 dose, then detrermine dosing interval for a maximum of either 1 or 2 further doses based on renal function (see Tables 1 and 2) |

IV, intravenous; QUIAC, Quality Use of Antimicrobials in Intensive Care.

**Table 6: Management of Trauma Orthopedics and Multitrauma**

| Regimen | Drug | Dose |
|---|---|---|
| Orthopedics non-elective trauma | Cefazolin<br><br>or | 2 g IV 8 hourly |
| Orthopedics non-elective trauma | Vancomycin | 1.5 g IV 12 hourly (adjust initial dosage for renal function, and subsequent doses to achieve therapeutic range) |

IV, intravenous.

**Table 7: Management of Suspected Fungal Sepsis**

| Regimen | Drug | Dose |
|---|---|---|
| Azole naïve, no prior isolates of *Candida glabrate* or *C. kruzei* | • Fluconazole<br><br>or<br><br>• Amphotericin B<br><br>or<br><br>• Caspofungin | • 800 mg IV first dose and then 400 mg IV daily<br><br>or<br><br>• 0.5 –1 mg/kg IV daily<br><br>or<br><br>• 70 mg IV first dose, then 50 mg IV daily |

IV, intravenous.

**Table 8: Predetermine Duration of Antibiotic Therapy based on the Infectious Diseases Society of America Guidelines**

| Site of infection | Duration of antibiotic therapy (days) |
| --- | --- |
| **Lung infection** | |
| CAP due to *S. pneumoniae* | 8 |
| VAP | 8 |
| VAP and immunodepression | 14 |
| Pneumonia due to *Legionella pneumophila* | 21 |
| Pneumonia with lung necrosis | ≥28 |
| **Intra-abdominal infections** | |
| Community peritonitis | <8 |
| Postoperative peritonitis | 14 |
| **CNS infections** | |
| Meningococcemia | 5–8 |
| Meningitis due to *S. pneumoniae* | 10–14 |
| Postoperative meningitis due to *S. epidermidis* or *Enterobacteriaceae* | 14 |
| Meningitis due to *Listeria monocytogenes* | 21 |
| Postoperative meningitis due to *S. aureus* or *P. aeruginosa* | 21 |
| Brain abscess | ≥28 |
| **Catheter-related bacteremia** | |
| *S. epidermidis* or *Enterobacteriaceae* | <8 |
| *S. aureus*/*Candida* species (uncomplicated) | 14 |
| *S. aureus* (complicated) | ≥28 |

CAP, community-acquired pneumonia; VAP, ventilator-associated pneumonia; CNS, central nervous system.

Given this wide plethora of reasons, cutting down on antibiotic usage could be done without harming health outcomes. Actually this could improve both short-term and long-term outcomes in our country.

## *Spread of Multidrug Resistance*

Even though the emergence of multidrug resistance is ascribed to excessive and indiscriminate antibiotic usage (>60% of patients in intensive care have received antibiotics during this stay),[22] the actual epidemiology of MDR is much more complex and multifactorial. Over the years, we have realized that there are certain antibiotics which seem to breed higher resistance patterns, e.g., third-generation cephalosporins, vancomycin, imipenem, and intravenous (IV) fluoroquinolones.[23,24]

On the other hand, there are other antibiotics (e.g., colistin) which have been used for decades and still barely cause any resistance.

Bonten and Mascini recognized four main forces behind the emergence and for this spread of MDR microorganisms:[25]

- Induction of resistant strains
- Selection of resistance strains
- Introduction of resistance strains
- Dissemination of resistance strains.

These relative forces should be considered when trying to tackle the antimicrobial resistance. This is especially so because all microorganisms have their own mechanisms and flexibility to become resistant depending on their ideal microenvironment.[25]

### Induction of Resistant Strains

Resistance of susceptible bacteria can occur during antimicrobial treatment, e.g., by mutation.[25] Quinolones and cephalosporins resistance in *Enterobacter* species may arise through this mechanism.

### Selection of Resistance Strains

Antimicrobial therapy may promote the growth of a pre-existing resistant bacteria.[25] It is important to maintain the nonpathogenic (anaerobic) flora, e.g., in the gastrointestinal tract, to prevent the overgrowth of Gram-negative MDR microorganisms.[25]

### Introduction of Resistance Strains

The expanding flora of MDR microorganisms in the community also results in a rise of MDR microorganisms in ICU. This is especially true for species such as MRSA and vancomycin-resistant enterococcus (VRE).[25] Healthcare workers are often carriers but can also be vectors (cross-contamination).[25,26] Also, an increasing number of patients are often colonized by bacteria at the time of ICU admission.[25] When colonization pressure with resistant strains is above a certain level, the risk of cross-contamination is extremely high and very difficult to overcome (inoculum effect).[23]

### Dissemination of Resistant Strains

Dissemination of resistant strains in all microorganisms is due to suboptimal infection control which also facilitates the spread of MDR microorganisms.[25]

## Important Resistant Pathogens

Over the past decade, there has been a paradigm shift of resistant microorganisms from Gram-positive to the Gram-negative variety. This is especially so because of scarcity of new antibiotics against Gram-negative microorganisms.[27] MRSA and VRE are the most important Gram-positive microorganisms in ICU.[27,28] The expanding numbers of Gram-negative bacteria is mainly due to the rapid increase of extended-spectrum beta-lactamases in *Klebsiella pneumoniae, E. coli,* and *Proteus mirabilis*; high-level third-generation cephalosporins β-lactamases resistance among *Enterobacter* species and *Citrobacter* species; and MDR *P. aeruginosa, Acinetobacter* species, and *Stenotrophomonas maltophilia.*[28] Together with this Gram-negative bugs, there has been the emergence of other types of infections which have all certificate to treat, e.g., anaerobic *Clostridium* species and fungal infections.

## PREVENTION OF INFECTIONS IN INTENSIVE CARE UNIT

Simple measures to prevent infection and pathogen cross-transmission assume significance considering the huge expenses incurred in terms of patient morbidity and mortality as well as the indirect costs involved in treating a resistant infection. A summary of the recommendations made by the Centers for Disease Control and Prevention (CDC) is given below.

Preventing central venous catheter infection:

- Educate personnel about catheter insertion and care
- Use chlorhexidine to prepare the insertion site
- Use maximal barrier precautions during catheter insertion
- Consolidate insertion supplies (e.g., in an insertion kit or cart)
- Use a checklist to enhance adherence to the bundle
- Empower nurses to halt insertion if asepsis is breached
- Cleanse patients daily with chlorhexidine
- Ask daily: is the catheter needed? Remove catheter if not needed or used.

Prevention of VAP:

- Elevate head end of bed to 30–45°
- Decontaminate oropharynx regularly with chlorhexidine
- Give "sedation vacation" and assess readiness to extubate daily
- Use peptic ulcer disease prophylaxis
- Use deep vein thrombosis prophylaxis (unless contraindicated).

Prevention of UTIs:

- Place bladder catheters only when absolutely needed (e.g., to relieve obstruction), not solely for the provider's convenience
- Use aseptic technique for catheter insertion and urinary tract instrumentation
- Minimize manipulation or opening of drainage systems
- Ask daily: is the catheter needed? Remove catheter if not needed.

Prevention of surgical site infections:

- Choose a surgeon wisely
- Administer prophylactic antibiotics within 1 hour before surgery; discontinue within 24 hours
- Limit any hair removal to the time of surgery; use clippers or do not remove hair at all.
- Prepare surgical site with chlorhexidine-alcohol.
- Maintain normal perioperative blood glucose levels (cardiac surgery patients)
- Maintain perioperative normothermia (colorectal surgery patients).

Prevention of pathogen cross-transmission:

- Cleanse hands with alcohol hand rub before and after all contacts with patients or their environments.

Empiric treatment of sick "immunocompromised" patient (febrile neutropenia empiric treatment):

- Neutropenic patients may present without fever, however, a patient receiving chemotherapy, whether known to be neutropenic or not, who presents with fever, chills, rigors, or unwell should receive empiric antibiotic therapy without waiting for the results of investigations to become available
- Consider previous antimicrobial exposure and prior microbiology to guide empiric selection
- Consultation with the patient's hematologist or oncologist is recommended.

## CONCLUSION: POTENTIAL SOLUTIONS

The pipeline for new antibiotics is almost dry. Hence it becomes double important to ensure that we use our existing resources prudently to slow down the rising problem of MDR. The CDC recommends four different strategies for this: (i) prevent infections; (ii) diagnose and treat infections; (iii) prudent and rational use of antimicrobials; and (iv) prevent transmission. The only way to achieve this would be for the medical professional to join hands with the policy makers, hospital administrators, and the patients to minimize antibiotic usage. Antibiotic stewardship to optimize antibiotic usage for therapy and for prophylaxis would be cornerstone of this program. A team approach which includes the physician, an intensivist, nurse, infectious disease specialist, and a microbiologist should join hands in implementing "packages of interventions or care bundles" rather than "single strategies" in preventing infections. While these strategies are not evidence based, they are definitely going to be more likely in control and prevention of infections.

---

### Editor's Comment

*Infections are common in an intensive care unit (ICU) set up and, therefore, antibiotics are the most frequently prescribed drugs for patients admitted to any ICUs. Incidentally, ICU infections more commonly result from multidrug resistant organisms. On the other hand, there is great concern about the indiscriminate and excessive use of antimicrobial agents which promote the development of antibiotic resistance. Infection prevention and control is therefore crucial. Programs designed to encourage appropriate prescriptions in ICUs are important in treatment, prevention of antibiotic resistance, and cost containment. Antibiotic stewardship to optimize antibiotic usage for therapy and prophylaxis constitutes the cornerstone of such a program.*

***Surinder K Jindal***

---

## REFERENCES


1. Tabah A, Koulenti D, Laupland K, Misset B, Valles J, Bruzzi de Carvalho F, et al. Characteristics and determinants of outcome of hospital-acquired bloodstream infections in intensive care units: the EUROBACT International Cohort Study. *Intensive Care Med.* 2012;38:1930-45.
2. World Health Organization. World Health Statistics 2011. France; 2011.
3. Mathew JL. Pneumococcal vaccination in developing countries: where does science end and commerce begin? *Vaccine.* 2009;27:4247-51.
4. Levine OS, Cherian T. Pneumococcal vaccination for Indian children. *Indian Pediatr.* 2007;44:491-6.
5. Austin DJ, Kristinsson KG, Anderson RM. The relationship between the volume of antimicrobial consumption in human communities and the frequency of resistance. *Proc Natl Acad Sci USA.* 1999;96:1152-6.
6. Laxminarayan R, Malani A, Howard D, Smith DL. Extending the cure: policy responses to the growing threat of antibiotic resistance. Resources for the Future (RFF) Report. Washington, DC; 2007. [online] Available from: http://www.rff.org/Publications/Pages/PublicationDetails.aspx?PublicationID=9575. [Accessed August, 2015].
7. Fry DE. Fever in the ICU. In: Marino PL, Sutin KM (Eds). The ICU Book, 3rd edition. Philadelphia, PA: Lippincott Williams and Wilkins; 2008.
8. Kotwani A, Holloway K. Trends in antibiotic use among outpatients in New Delhi, India. *BMC Infect Dis.* 2011;11:99.
9. Yong D, Toleman MA, Giske CG, Cho HS, Sundman K, Lee K, et al. Characterization of a new metallo-beta-lactamase gene, bla(NDM-1), and a novel erythromycin esterase gene carried on a unique genetic structure in Klebsiella pneumoniae sequence type 14 from India. *Antimicrob Agents Chemother.* 2009;53:5046-54.

10. Deshpande P, Rodrigues C, Shetty A, Kapadia F, Hedge A, Soman R. New Delhi metallo-beta-lactamase (NDM-1) in Enterobacteriaceae: treatment options with carbapenems compromised. *J Assoc Physicians India*. 2010;58:147-9.

11. Holloway K, Mathai E, Sorensen TL, Gray A. Community-based surveillance of antimicrobial use and resistance in resource-constrained settings. US Agency for International Development Report on five pilot projects. Geneva: World Health Organization; 2009.

12. Thomas K, Lalitha MK, Arora NK, Das B, Awasthi S, Amita J, et al. Invasive bacterial infectious surveillance II (IBIS 2). Final report. Vellore; [online] Available from: http://www.inclentrust.org/resources/iphid/iidi/Annex 1-IBISI 2final.pdf. [Accessed August, 2015].

13. Mehta A, Rosenthal VD, Mehta Y, Chakravarthy M, Todi SK, Sen N, et al. Device-associated nosocomial infection rates in intensive care units of seven Indian cities. Findings of the International Nosocomial Infection Control Consortium (INICC). *J Hosp Infect*. 2007;67:168-74.

14. Kotwani A, Roy Chaudhury R, Holloway K. Conference paper: prescribing antibiotics for acute respiratory tract infections by primary care physicians in New Delhi, India. International Society of Pharmacoeconomics and Outcomes Research; 2010.

15. Kumar R, Indira K, Rizvi A, Rizvi T, Jeyaseelan L. Antibiotic prescribing practices in primary and secondary health care facilities in Uttar Pradesh, India. *J Clin Pharm Ther*. 2008;33:625-34.

16. Kotwani A, Wattal C, Katewa S, Joshi PC, Holloway K. Factors influencing primary care physicians to prescribe antibiotics in Delhi, India. *Fam Pract*. 2010;27:684-90.

17. Sivagnanam G, Thirumalaikolundusubramanian P, Mohanasundaram J, Raaj AA, Namasivayam K, Rajaram S. A survey on current attitude of practicing physicians upon usage of antimicrobial agents in southern part of India. *MedGenMed*. 2004;6:1.

18. Dua V, Kunin CM, White LV. The use of antimicrobial drugs in Nagpur, India. A window on medical care in a developing country. *Soc Sci Med*. 1994;38:717-24.

19. Kotwani A, Wattal C, Joshi PC, Holloway K. Irrational use of antibiotics and role of the pharmacist: an insight from a qualitative study in New Delhi, India. *J Clin Pharm Ther*. 2011;37(3):308-12.

20. Delhi Society for Promotion of Rational Use of Drugs. (WHO/SEARO). Promoting awareness amongst school children on rational use of drugs. Delhi; 2009.

21. Sharma R, Verma U, Sharma CL, Kapoor B. Self-medication among urban population of Jammu city. *Indian J Pharmacol*. 2005;37:37-45.

22. Borg MA. Bed occupancy and overcrowding as determinant factors in the incidence of MRSA infections within general ward settings. *J Hosp Infect*. 2003;54:316-8.

23. Carlet J, Ben Ali A, Tabah A, Willems V, Philippart F, Chafine A, et al. Multidrug resistant infections in the ICU: mechanisms, prevention and treatment. In: Kuhlen R, Moreno R, Ranieri VM, Rhodes A (Eds). 25 Years of Progress and Innovation in Intensive Care Medicine, 1st edition. Berlin, Germany: Medizinisch Wissenschaftliche Verlagsgesellschaft; 2007. pp. 199-211.

24. Clark NM, Hershberger E, Zervosc MJ, Lynch JP 3rd. Antimicrobial resistance among gram-positive organisms in the intensive care unit. *Curr Opin Crit Care*. 2003;9:403-12.

25. Bonten MJ, Mascini EM. The hidden faces of the epidemiology of antibiotic resistance. *Intensive Care Med*. 2003;29:1-2.

26. Salgado CD, O'Grady N, Farr BM. Prevention and control of antimicrobial-resistant infections in intensive care patients. *Crit Care Med*. 2005;33:2373-82.

27. Boucher HW, Talbot GH, Bradley JS, Edwards JE, Gilbert D, Rice LB, et al. Bad bugs, no drugs: no ESKAPE! An update from the Infectious Diseases Society of America. *Clin Infect Dis*. 2009;48:1-12.

28. Jones RN. Resistance patterns among nosocomial pathogens: trends over the past few years. *Chest*. 2001;119:397S-404S.

# WORLD CLINICS
## Statement of Purpose

The streams of medicine and surgery are evolving constantly at a rapid pace, creating a need for the healthcare professionals to continuously update their knowledge base and skills. This is necessary to offer their patients the best 'real world' treatment options based on current concepts, status, and trends, reflecting the achievements of evidence-based medicine. This pace of advances in medicine is a compelling reason for the physicians and surgeons to seek information through multiple resources, such as journals, workshops and conferences.

WORLD CLINICS are periodicals of evidence-based reviews  proposed as a source of comprehensive, state-of-the art reviews written by experts representing the global academia under the mentorship of an Editor-in-Chief. The comments by the 'Guest Editor' (or Editor-in-Chief) given at the end of each article/chapter would be representative of their clinical experience. Each issue of "WORLD CLINICS Pulmonary and Critical Care Medicine" would focus on a single theme covering topics that are relevant to clinical understanding and decision-making.  Each topic would be developed to reflect the current evidence, research, existing guidelines and recommendations as well the clinical experience of experts.

## Objectives

- Provide up-to-date reviews on disease management, technique, procedure, or technology.
- Help enhance knowledge and skill for application in clinical practice.
- To aid use of evidence in decision-making for improved patient care.
- To help select best treatment options and overcome treatment challenges.

## Target Readers

WORLD CLINICS are meant for practicing physicians, fellows, and postgraduate students, who plan to keep abreast with the current best-evidence clinical practices that are recommended and followed by experts globally.

## Periodicity

WORLD CLINICS Pulmonary and Critical Care Medicine will be released with a frequency of two issues in a year.

## Themes

Each subject area of WORLD CLINICS will cover themes on any of the following:

1. A disease or a disorder (e.g., Pneumonia) OR
2. An organ or an anatomical region (e.g., Wrist, in WORLD CLINICS  Orthopedics) OR
3. A technique or a treatment approach (e.g., Various methods for the treatment of CTEV, in WORLD CLINICS  Orthopedics) OR
4. A special population group (e.g., Management of HIV infected children patients in WORLD CLINICS Pediatrics) OR
5. A technology (e.g., 3D Ultrasound in diagnosis of gynecological abnormalities in WORLD CLINICS Obstetrics and Gynecology)

# WORLD CLINICS
## Manuscript Guidelines for Authors

## General Guidelines

- Manuscripts must be typed in double-space including all text, references, tables, and figure legends, and should be sent in a single word file.
- For any copyright work, the necessary permissions must be obtained by the author and sent along with the manuscript. These permissions apply to any borrowed, modified, or adapted text, tables, or figures.
- For any production-quality artwork (images, illustrations, etc.) please see the guidelines under images.
- Acknowledgments or disclosures, if required, should be cited before the references.

## Author Credits

- Should be in the first page.
- Each author's name, degree, academic or professional affiliation, city, and state (or country).
- E-mail address, mailing address, and telephone number of each co-author.
- If more than one author, mention the corresponding author.
- Please supply 4–6 keywords which will be used to optimize search results.

## Subheads

The format for article's headings and subheadings is as follows:
'A' head: All caps, bold.
'B' head: Title case (upper/lower), bold.
'C' head: Title case (upper/lower), bold, italics.
'D' head: Title case (upper lower), normal, Roman.
'E' head: Sentence case (initial letter capital), italics, run in.

## References

- References must be cited sequentially only at the end of the manuscript in the order as they appear in the text.
- Follow the Vancouver style for the references, using the Index Medicus abbreviations for journals that are indexed; if a journal is not indexed, use full name.
- If there are more than six authors, cite first six and add "et al.," e.g., Lacasse Y, Selman M, Costabel U, Dalphin JC, Ando M, Morell F, et al. Clinical diagnosis of hypersensitivity pneumonitis. *Am J Respir Crit Care Med.* 2003;168:952-8.

## Images

- There is generally no restriction on number of boxes, tables, or images, but keep them to a minimum necessary.
- A maximum of two hand-drawn illustrations and maximum of two algorithms are allowed.
- Medium for delivery of photographs: Individual TIFF or JPEG files each at a resolution no lower than 300 dpi (118 pixels/cm) when viewed at 100 mm width.
- The images and illustrations can also be in full color.